NUC

ENGLISH FOR SCIENCE AND TECHNOLOGY

MEDICINE

Tony O'Brien
with
Jeffrey Jameson
and
David Kirwan

Series Editors
Martin Bates and Tony Dudley-Evans
Science Adviser to the Series
Arthur Godman C. Chem., MRIC

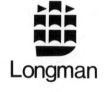

Longman

Longman Group UK Limited
Longman House, Burnt Mill, Harlow,
Essex CM20 2JE, England
and Associated Companies throughout the world.

First published 1979
Tenth impression 1991

Produced by Longman Group (FE) Ltd
Printed in Hong Kong

ISBN 0-582-51307-3

Acknowledgements

We wish to thank Dr John Nimmo, B.Sc. (Hons), M.B., Ch.B., F.R.C.P., Consultant Physician, Eastern General Hospital, Edinburgh for his helpful comments on the medical content of this book.

T.O'B., J.J. and D.K.

The publishers are grateful to the following for permission to reproduce copyright material:
Baillière Tindall and the author, Dr P. E. C. Manson Bahr for adapted extracts from *Tropical Diseases* by Dr Manson Bahr; Churchill Livingstone and the editor, Dr J. Macleod for adapted extracts from *Davidson's Principles and Practices of Medicine* 12th Edition; J. B. Lippincott Company for an adapted extract from *Pathologic Physiology* 9th Edition by E. M. Greisheimer and M. P. Wiedmann.

Contents

A Guide to Verbalisation

Numbers

285	two hundred and eighty five
3150	three thousand one hundred and fifty
5038	five thousand and thirty eight
36·3	thirty six point three
36·36	thirty six point three six
0	zero/nought
0·75	zero/nought point seven five
0·05	nought point nought five
$\frac{1}{3}$	a third (one third)
$\frac{1}{4}$	a quarter (one quarter)
$\frac{1}{2}$	a half
15/20	fifteen over twenty (fifteen twentieths)
<0·4	less than nought point four
>1·0	more than one point nought
11×10^9	eleven times ten to the power of nine (ten to the ninth)
c. 70	about seventy
1:4	one to four

Others (see also Unit 4, ex.1)

37·2°C	thirty seven point two degrees Centigrade
104°F	a hundred and four degrees Fahrenheit
26·5%	twenty six point five per cent
120/80 mm/Hg	one twenty over eighty millimetres of mercury
mmol/l	millimoles per litre
ng	nanogram (a thousand millionth of a gram)
$11 \times 6 \times 3$	eleven by six by three
$C = \frac{1}{3}B$	C equals one third (of) B
H_2CO_3	/eɪtʃ tuː siː əʊ θriː/
$Na(HCO_3)_2$	/en eɪ eɪtʃ siː əʊ θriː tuː/

Years

1900	nineteen hundred
1906	nineteen oh six
1984	nineteen eighty four

Unit 1   Shapes and Properties

Section 1   Presentation

1. Look at these diagrams:

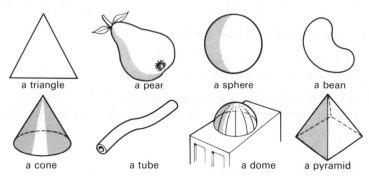

a triangle   a pear   a sphere   a bean

a cone   a tube   a dome   a pyramid

Now look at this diagram and complete the sentences:

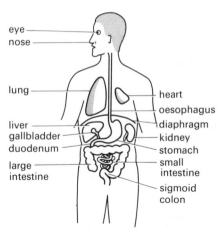

Example: The heart *is shaped like* a cone.
a) The eye is shaped like ....
b) The diaphragm ....
c) The kidneys ....
d) The lungs ....
e) The gallbladder ....
f) The oesophagus ....
g) The liver ....
h) The nose ....

2. Look at this example:

The gallbladder is a *pear-shaped* organ.

Complete the sentences with *one* of these words:

kidneys   oesophagus   duodenum   dome-shaped   S-shaped

a) The diaphragm is a ...... organ.
b) The sigmoid colon is an ...... organ.
c) The ...... is a C-shaped tube.
d) The ...... are bean-shaped organs.

7

3. Make six sentences from this table:

The liver is	conical in shape.
The eye is	a long, tubular organ.
The nose is	triangular in shape.
The kidneys are	a small, spherical organ.
The heart is	pyramidal in shape.
The small intestine is	bean-shaped organs.

4. From exercises 1–3 find two ways of describing:

    a) the heart; the eye; the liver
    b) the kidneys; the gallbladder; the diaphragm

Now describe each of the following in two different ways:
    c) the oesophagus; the lungs; the duodenum; the sigmoid colon; the small
    intestine

Section 2　Development

5. Look and read:

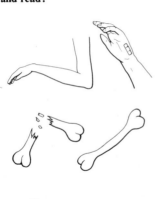
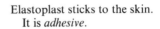

Elastoplast sticks to the skin.
    It is *adhesive*.

The skin can bend into many shapes.
    It is *flexible*.

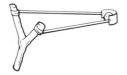

Bones cannot bend.
    They are *rigid*.

Some tissues can be stretched and then will
return to their original shape.
    They are *elastic*.

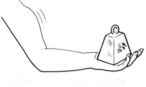

Some organs can stretch or contract by the
use of muscles.
    They are *muscular*.

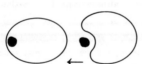

Some cells can eat bacteria and destroy
them.
    They are *phagocytic*.

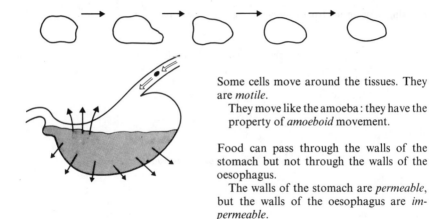

Some cells move around the tissues. They are *motile*.

They move like the amoeba: they have the property of *amoeboid* movement.

Food can pass through the walls of the stomach but not through the walls of the oesophagus.

The walls of the stomach are *permeable*, but the walls of the oesophagus are *impermeable*.

Now look at this diagram of blood vessels:

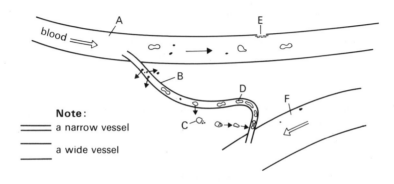

Note:
≡ a narrow vessel

─ a wide vessel

Complete these sentences and match them with A to F in the diagram:

a) Arteries are long, tubular blood vessels which can bend and stretch, i.e. they are ...... and ....
b) Some cells and molecules can pass through capillary walls. In other words capillaries are ....
c) Some white blood cells (leucocytes) can destroy bacteria, i.e. leucocytes are ....
d) Platelets are very small particles which stick together to stop bleeding, i.e. they are ....
e) Red blood cells (erythrocytes) can bend to get through narrow blood vessels and then spring back into shape. In other words erythrocytes ....
f) Blood cells cannot pass through artery walls. This means that arteries ....
g) Leucocytes can pass through capillary walls. This means that capillary walls are ...... to leucocytes.
h) The leucocytes can move around in the tissues, or, in other words, they ....
i) Veins are wide blood vessels with some muscle tissue in their walls, i.e. veins ....
j) Erythrocytes can not usually pass through capillary walls. In other words, capillary walls are usually ....

6. Using information from exercise 5, complete these tables:

	flexible	phagocytic	motile	adhesive
erythrocytes		×	×	×
leucocytes	√			
platelets	√	×	×	

	permeable	impermeable	muscular	elastic
arteries			√	
capillaries			×	×
veins		√		×

Read these:

> *Both* erythrocytes *and* leucocytes are flexible.
> *Neither* erythrocytes *nor* leucocytes are adhesive.
>
> Leucocytes are phagocytic $\begin{cases}but\\whereas\end{cases}$ erythrocytes are not.
>
> Leucocytes are phagocytic. Erythrocytes, $\begin{cases}however\\on\ the\ other\ hand\end{cases}$, are not.
>
> Leucocytes can pass through capillary walls, but veins are impermeable to leucocytes.

Complete these sentences:

a) Both arteries and ...... impermeable.
b) Arteries are elastic blood vessels but ....
c) Capillaries have very thin walls whereas ...... muscular walls.
d) Capillaries are permeable to .... Erythrocytes, on the other hand, ...
e) Leucocytes can pass through the walls of capillaries. Arteries, however ....
f) Neither ...... are phagocytic.
g) Platelets are ...... erythrocytes are not.
h) ...... do not have the ...... of amoeboid movement. Leucocytes ...... can ...... tissues.
i) Skin is .... Bone ...... is rigid.

Section 3 Reading

7. Read the passage and label these diagrams:

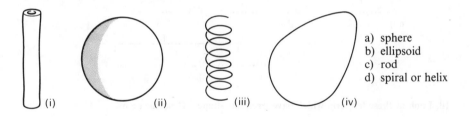

a) sphere
b) ellipsoid
c) rod
d) spiral or helix

Bacteria

Bacteria are very small, unicellular organisms. Although there are thousands of
different species of bacteria, the individual organisms have one of three general
forms: ellipsoidal, or spherical; cylindrical or rod-like; and spiral or helicoidal.

The first type are called *cocci* (singular, *coccus*). They are nearly all spherical
5 or ellipsoidal, but there are some exceptions. The gonococcus and meningo-
coccus, for example, are coffee-bean shaped (e.g. *Neisseria meningitidis*), while
the pneumococcus is slightly elongated, so that one end tapers a little (e.g.
Diplococcus pneumoniae, in which the ends of each pair of cells are bluntly
pointed).

10 The cylindrical bacteria are known as *bacilli* (singular, *bacillus*). Some of these
are long and slender (e.g. *Clostridium sporogenes*) while others are short and
thick (e.g. *Bacillus megaterium*). The sides may be more or less parallel to each
other or the cell may be thicker in the centre and taper toward the end.

Spiral forms include rods with just enough curvature to give the organism a
15 curved or comma shape (Vibrio), longer rigid rods with several curves or spirals
(Spirillum) and long flexible organisms with several or many spirals (spiro-
chaetes).

8. Read the passage again and label the following bacteria:

Diplococcus pneumoniae   *Vibrio comma*
Neisseria meningitidis   *Spirillum volutans*
Clostridium sporogenes   *Spirochaeta stenostrepta*
Bacillus megaterium

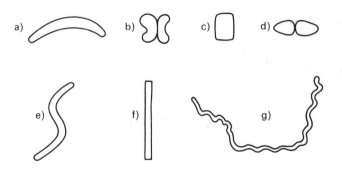

9. Summarise the types of bacteria mentioned in the passage by completing this classification diagram. Give an example of each type:

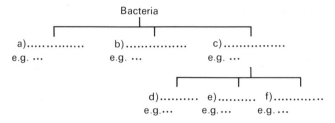

Bacteria

a)..............   b)...............   c)...............
e.g. ···   e.g. ···   e.g. ···

d)..........   e)..........   f).............
e.g.···   e.g.···   e.g.···

10. Look at these bacteria which have irregular shapes. Describe them.

    a) *Saprospira sp.*   b) *Caulobacter sp.*   c) *Streptomyces sp.*

  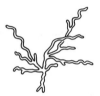

Section 4   Listening

11. Listen to the passage and label these diagrams:

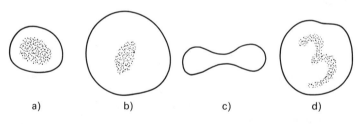

a)   b)   c)   d)

erythrocytes   polymorphonuclear leucocytes
lymphocytes   monocytes

Now complete this classification diagram:

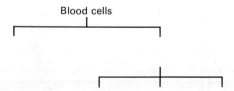

Blood cells

12. Listen to the passage again and choose the correct word(s) in these sentences:

    a) Erythrocytes are flexible/rigid and concave/convex.

    b) Polymorphonuclear leucocytes are adhesive/phagocytic and amoeboid/ elastic.

    c) Monocytes are permeable/phagocytic.

13. Describe the four types of cells, using the diagrams in exercise 11 and the information in exercise 12 to help you:

Unit 2 Location

Section 1 Presentation

1. Look and read:

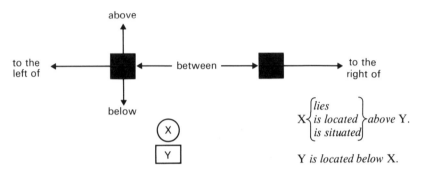

Now complete the sentences below this diagram:

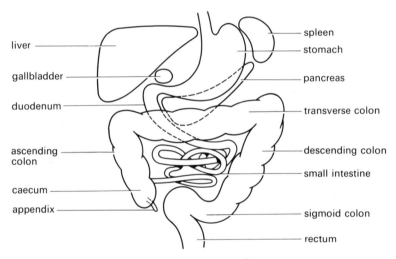

N.B.   RIGHT (of the body)   LEFT

Some organs of the abdomen

    a) The stomach lies between the liver and ....
    b) ...... is situated above the descending colon.
    c) The small intestine is located between ...... and ....
    d) ...... is to the right of the spleen.
    e) The transverse colon lies ...... the stomach.
    f) The stomach is ...... the liver.
    g) The liver is ...... the ascending colon.
    h) The pancreas is located to the left of ....
    i) ...... is situated below the small intestine.
    j) The gallbladder lies below ...... and ...... the duodenum.

2. Look and read:

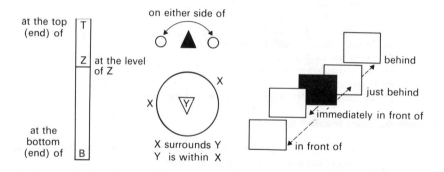

Now complete the sentences below these diagrams:

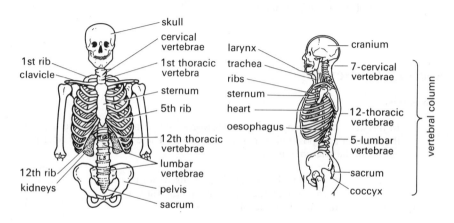

The skeleton (from the front)   The skeleton (from the left side)

a) The heart is situated immediately behind ....
b) ...... lies just in front of the vertebral column.
c) The cervical vertebrae are located at the top end of ....
d) ...... are situated at the bottom end of the vertebral column.
e) ...... lie on either side of the vertebral column.
f) The top of the right kidney is at the level of ....
g) The ribs ...... the heart.

3. Read this example:

sternum – heart

Q. Where *does* the sternum *lie*
    Where *is* the sternum *located* } *in relation to* the heart?

A. The sternum lies *just in front of* the heart.

15

Ask and answer similar questions:

    a) sacrum – coccyx
    b) rectum – large intestine
    c) vertebral column – heart
    d) larynx – vertebral column and trachea
    e) top of left kidney – 11th rib
    f) liver – diaphragm and stomach
    g) lungs – ribs
    h) duodenum – liver, transverse colon and pancreas

4. Name the organs described here:

    a) This is a triangular organ which lies immediately in front of the oesophagus at the level of the 4th to 6th cervical vertebrae.
    b) This is a short, curved tube which is located immediately behind and below a wide tubular section of the intestine.
    c) This is a flexible organ which lies in the middle of the abdomen just below and behind the stomach, and tapers up to the left.
    d) This is a wide tubular section of the intestine which is situated at the bottom end of the ascending colon.

Section 2   Development

5. Read this:

In the study of anatomy many special words and phrases are used to describe the location and position of parts of the body. These terms always refer to a person in the anatomic position.

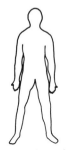

A person who is standing, facing forward, with arms at the sides and palms turned forward, is in the *anatomic position.*

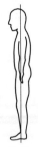

A *coronal* (or *frontal*) *plane* passes through the body from top to bottom and divides it into front and back sections.

Anterior (or *ventral*) ⎫ means nearer the ⎰ *front.*
Posterior (or *dorsal*) ⎭   ⎱ *back.*

Example: The heart is posterior to the sternum.
               a) The heart is anterior to ....

A *transverse* (or *horizontal*) *plane* divides
the body into upper and lower sections.

$\left.\begin{array}{l}Superior\\Inferior\end{array}\right\}$ means nearer to the $\left\{\begin{array}{l}head.\\feet.\end{array}\right.$

Example: The stomach is superior to the transverse colon.
b) ...... is inferior to the small intestine.

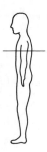

The *midsagittal plane* passes through
the middle of the body from top to bottom
and divides it into right and left sections.

A *sagittal plane* is any other plane which
divides the body into right and left sections,
but does not pass through the middle of the body.

$\left.\begin{array}{l}Medial\\Lateral\end{array}\right\}$ means $\left\{\begin{array}{l}nearer\ to\\farther\ from\end{array}\right\}$ the midline of the body.

Example: The kidneys are lateral to the vertebral column.
c) The heart is medial to ....

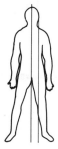

$\left.\begin{array}{l}Proximal\\Distal\end{array}\right\}$ means $\left\{\begin{array}{l}nearer\ to\\farther\ from\end{array}\right\}$ the origin of a part.

Example: A is the proximal end of the femur.
d) B is ....
e) The shin is distal to the thigh.
f) The ankle is proximal to ....

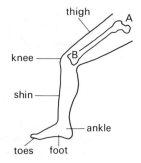

17

6. Label these diagrams:

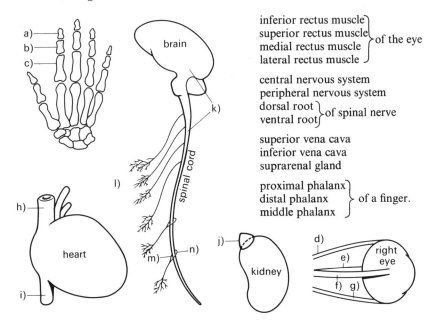

inferior rectus muscle ⎫
superior rectus muscle ⎬ of the eye
medial rectus muscle ⎪
lateral rectus muscle ⎭

central nervous system
peripheral nervous system
dorsal root ⎫ of spinal nerve
ventral root ⎭

superior vena cava
inferior vena cava
suprarenal gland

proximal phalanx ⎫
distal phalanx ⎬ of a finger.
middle phalanx ⎭

7. Look and read:

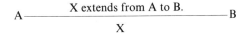

X extends from A to B.

The small intestine is a narrow tube which extends from the stomach to the colon. It has three parts: the duodenum, the jejunum and the ileum. The duodenum lies on the posterior abdominal wall. It extends from the stomach to the duodenojejunal flexure.

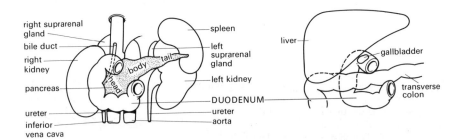

Anterior aspects of the duodenum with related organs

The superior (1st) part of the duodenum is related posteriorly to the pancreas and the common bile duct. Anteriorly it is in contact with the liver and gallbladder. Inferiorly it rests on the pancreas.

Now complete the description of the location of the duodenum:

The descending (2nd) part is related posteriorly to .... Anteriorly it is crossed by .... Above the transverse colon it is in contact with ......, and ...... with coils of small intestine. On its left lie .... The horizontal (3rd) part lies below ......, and posteriorly it crosses, from right to left, the .... The ascending (4th) part lies to the left of the vertebral column.

8. Read this:

One of these statements is false. Which one?

Posteriorly the head of the pancreas is in contact with the inferior vena cava.
The head of the pancreas is in contact *posteriorly* with the inferior vena cava.
The head of the pancreas is in contact with the inferior vena cava *posteriorly*.

The first two sentences mean that the posterior part of the head of the pancreas is in contact with the inferior vena cava – which is true. But the third sentence has the opposite meaning, that the head of the pancreas is in contact with the posterior part of the inferior vena cava – which is false.

Say whether these statements are true or false. Correct the false ones.

a) Anteriorly the head of the pancreas is in contact with the inferior vena cava.
b) Posteriorly the bile duct is in contact with the inferior vena cava.
c) The pancreas lies medial to the ascending part of the duodenum.
d) Superiorly the head of the pancreas is in contact with the horizontal part of the duodenum.
e) The left ureter is medial to the ascending part of the duodenum.
f) The spleen lies anterosuperior to the left kidney.
g) The large blood vessels run medially to the ureters.
h) Posteriorly the head of the pancreas is in contact with the transverse colon.
i) The inferior surface of the body of the pancreas is related to the duodeno-jejunal flexure.
j) The transverse colon is related posteroinferiorly to the liver.

9. Look at the diagram of the blood supply in the pelvic area and name the arteries described here:

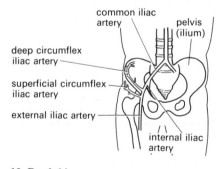

a) This artery descends from the common iliac artery into the pelvis, where it supplies the organs within the pelvis.
b) This artery passes outside the edge of the pelvis and passes on downwards into the leg.
c) This artery arises from the lateral side of the external iliac artery and supplies the inner pelvic wall.
d) This artery supplies the upper thigh and the outer parts of the pelvic wall.

10. Read this:

The aorta has many *visceral* and *parietal* branches. The *visceral* branches supply the organs (viscera) within the thoracic, abdominal and pelvic cavities, while the *parietal* branches supply the muscles and other tissues in the walls of the cavities.

Say whether these arteries are visceral or parietal branches:

Artery	(supplying)
a) gastric arteries	(stomach)
b) intercostal arteries	(muscles + tissues of rib cage)
c) mesenteric arteries	(intestines)
d) renal arteries	(kidneys)
e) phrenic arteries	(diaphragm)
f) median sacral artery	(posterior pelvic wall)

Section 3   Reading

11. Read the passage and label the diagram:

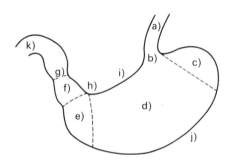

The stomach

This is a dilatation of the alimentary canal between the oesophagus and the duodenum. Although variable in size and shape it is usually J-shaped. The stomach is divided into a fundus, a body and a pyloric portion. It has anterior and posterior surfaces, and lesser and greater curvatures. The *fundus* is that part
5   above the level of the oesophageal opening (*cardiac orifice*). The body extends from the fundus to the *angular notch* (the lowest part of the lesser curvature) and the pyloric portion from the notch to the pyloric sphincter (*pylorus*) which separates the stomach from the duodenum. The pyloric part has two sections: a proximal dilated *pyloric antrum* and a distal tubular pyloric canal. The *lesser*
10 *curvature* is the upper medial border, which extends from the right of the oesophagus to the pylorus. The angular notch is near its lower end. The *greater curvature* extends from the left of the oesophagus around the fundus to the pylorus, forming the lateral border of the stomach.

Say whether the following sentences are true or false. Correct the false ones.

l)   The stomach is a tubular organ, like the other parts of the digestive system.
m) The stomach is situated medial to the oesophagus and duodenum.
n)   The fundus is superior to the cardiac orifice.
o)   The duodenum is distal to the pyloric canal.
p)   The angular notch is on the anterior surface of the stomach.

20

12. Look at the diagram and answer the questions:

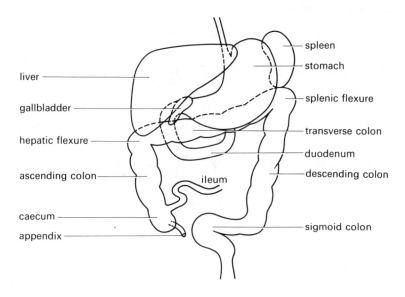

Anterior aspect of some organs of the abdomen

    a) What are the posterior relations of the transverse colon?
       (*Answer:* Posteriorly the transverse colon is related to ....)
    b) Where is the stomach in relation to the transverse colon?
       (*Answer:* The stomach is ...... to the transverse colon.)
    c) Where does the stomach lie in relation to the spleen?
    d) Where is the liver in relation to the colon?
    e) What are the anterosuperior relations of the transverse colon, from left to
       right?
    f) What are the relations of the spleen?
    g) Where does the appendix arise?
    h) What are the relations of the gallbladder?

13. Read this:

The ascending colon extends from the ileocaecal orifice to the right colic (hepatic)
flexure, which is in contact superiorly with the under-surface of the right lobe of
the liver. Posteriorly it lies on the lower part of the right kidney. Its anterior and
medial surfaces are in contact with coils of small intestine.

Write a similar passage about the descending colon. Begin like this:

The descending colon extends from ...... (which is ......) to .... Posteriorly
.... Its ...... surfaces are ....

Section 4 Listening

14. Look at the first diagram and listen to the three short passages. Write down the names of the organs being described:

(**Note:** one of the organs is not on the diagram.)

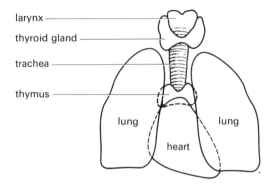

Anterior aspect of the thorax and neck

Look at the second diagram and listen to the first passage again.

Label the diagram with these names:

thyroid gland
isthmus
trachea
oesophagus

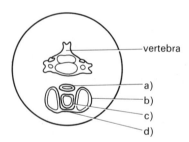

Transverse section of the neck at the level of the 6th cervical vertebra

15. Now read these sentences and say whether they are true or false. Correct the false statements.

a) (A) .... is situated inferior to the larynx.
b) It lies posterolateral to the trachea.
c) The isthmus crosses the trachea superiorly.
d) (B) .... lies immediately in front of the trachea.
e) It is posterosuperior to the heart.
f) It is situated in the lower part of the neck.
g) (C) .... is above and behind the stomach.
h) It has no fixed shape.
i) It is usually shaped like a long rod.
j) It does not have many blood vessels.

Unit 3   Structure

Section 1   Presentation

1. Look and read:

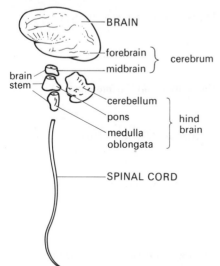

The nervous system *consists of* the central nervous system and the peripheral nervous system.

The central nervous system *is made up of* the brain and the spinal cord.

Both the spinal cord and the brain *are composed of* nerve cells and fibres.

The forebrain, the midbrain and the hind-brain *make up* the brain.

The pons, the cerebellum and the medulla oblongata *compose* the hindbrain.

The brain *contains* grey and white matter.

Now look at these diagrams and answer the questions:

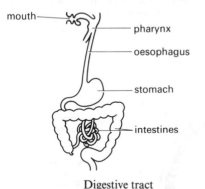

Digestive tract

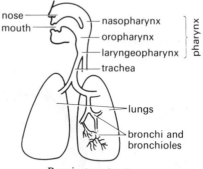

Respiratory tract

a) What is the brain stem composed of?
b) What composes the cerebrum?
c) What does the digestive tract consist of?
d) What are the intestines made up of? (two parts)
e) Which three organs make up the small intestine?
f) Of what parts is the large intestine composed?
g) What does the respiratory tract consist of?
h) What makes up the pharynx?
i) What do the lungs contain?
j) What does the skeletal system consist of?

23

2. Read this:

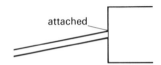

The body *is covered with* skin and hair.

The limbs *are attached to* the trunk.

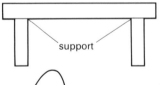

The body *is supported by* the legs.

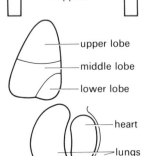

The lungs *are divided into* lobes.

Arteries *are filled with* blood.

The heart *is surrounded by* the lungs.

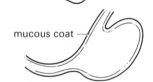

The stomach *is lined with* a mucous coat.

The thorax *is separated from* the abdomen *by* the diaphragm.

Look at this diagram:

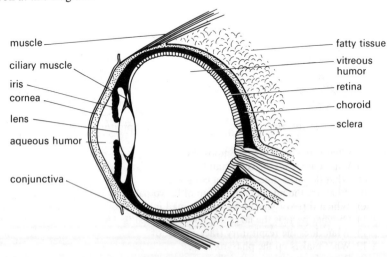

Horizontal section through the eyeball

Now complete these sentences with words from the list:

is covered by   is filled with   contains
is lined with   is surrounded by   divides
is supported by   is attached to   lines
                       is separated from

a) The biconvex lens ...... the cavity of the eyeball into two parts.
b) The posterior part ...... the jelly-like vitreous humor.
c) The anterior part ...... a watery fluid (aqueous humor).
d) The lens ...... the ciliary muscles.
e) The choroid ...... the retina.
f) The choroid ...... the sclera.
g) The sclera ...... the orbit (the bone surrounding the eye) by six small muscles.
h) The eye ...... fatty tissue.
i) The front of the eyeball ...... the conjunctiva.
j) The vitreous humour ...... the aqueous humor by the lens.

3. Look at the diagram and answer the questions:

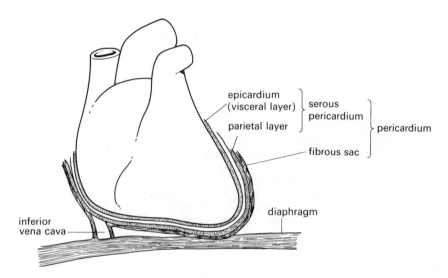

Covering of the heart

a) What is the heart covered by?
b) What does the pericardium consist of?
c) What is the fibrous sac attached to inferiorly?
d) What is the fibrous sac lined with?
e) What does the serous pericardium consist of?
f) What does the epicardium cover?
g) What is the heart filled with?
h) Into how many chambers is the heart divided?
i) What separates the heart from the lungs?

Section 2 Development

4. Look at this:

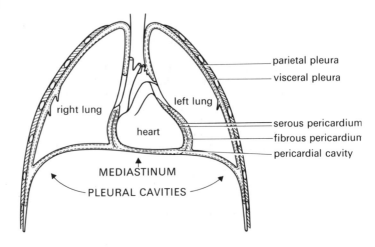

The cavities of the thorax and their linings

Complete the sentences with these words:

mediastinum	covers	is divided	are covered
pleural cavities	lines	is lined	are surrounded

a) The thorax ...... into three compartments.
b) ...... is the central compartment.
c) The mediastinum ...... by the pericardium.
d) The lateral compartments are known as ....
e) The lungs ...... by the pleura.
f) Parietal pleura ...... the outer walls of the cavity.
g) Visceral (pulmonary) pleura ...... the lungs.
h) All three compartments ...... by the ribs.

Now add one of these clauses to sentences (a) to (e), and write them out as a paragraph:

- which contains the heart, oesophagus, trachea, thymus and various blood vessels and nerves.
- which contain the lungs.
- which also surrounds the heart.
- which are called the mediastinum and the pleural cavities.
- which also lines the pleural cavities.

5. Read this and label the diagrams:

Tissue consists of living cells which are similar in structure and function, and non-living intercellular substance joining the cells together. Human tissue includes four main types: epithelial, connective, muscular and nervous tissue.

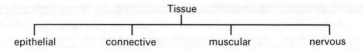

26

The tissue making up the outer layer of skin, known as the epidermis, is epithelial tissue, and so are the tissues lining systems such as the digestive, respiratory, urinary, etc. (i.e. systems opening onto the body surface).

Tissue consisting of one layer of cells is called simple epithelial and tissue consisting of more than one layer is known as stratified epithelial tissue. Epithelial tissue can also be classified according to the shape of the cells at the surface as squamous (flat), cubic or columnar.

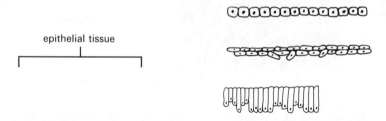

epithelial tissue

6. Look at this:

Tissue consists of living and non-living intercellular substance.
The intercellular substance joins tissue cells together.

We can also say: Tissue consists of living cells and non-living intercellular substance *which joins* the tissue cells together.

or: Tissue consists of living cells and non-living intercellular substance *joining* the tissue cells together.

Complete these sentences:

a) Epithelial tissue makes up ....
b) Epithelial tissue ...... the digestive system.
c) The respiratory system is a system which ....

Read this:

Simple epithelial tissue is epithelial tissue which consists of one layer of cells.

Now complete these definitions:

d) Stratified epithelial tissue is epithelial tissue which ....
e) Squamous epithelial tissue consists of cells which ....
f) Cubic epithelial tissue consists of ....
g) Columnar epithelial tissue ....

7. Look and read:

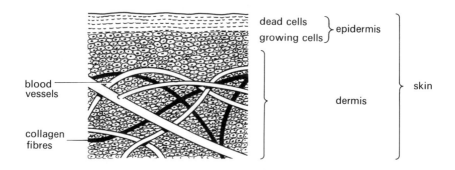

The skin, or cutis, is a membrane made up of two layers, and attached to the subcutaneous tissues by collagen fibres. The outer layer is the epidermis, composed of epithelial tissue developed from ectoderm. The epidermis has a deep layer of growing cells covered by a layer of dried dead cells. The inner layer is the dermis, composed of vascular connective tissue developed from embryonic mesoderm.

Read this:

The skin is a membrane. *The membrane is made* up of two layers.
or: The skin is a membrane *which is made* up of two layers.
or: The skin is a membrane *made* up of two layers. (composition)

Complete these:

a) ...... is attached to the subcutaneous tissues.
b) The epidermis ...... epithelial tissue. (composition)
c) The epithelial tissue of the epidermis ...... ectoderm. (origin)

Now write sentences about:

d) the composition of the deep layer of the epidermis.
e) the covering of the deep layer of the epidermis.
f) the composition of the dermis.
g) the origin of the dermis.

8. Look at this example:

thorax/large cavity/three compartments

The thorax is a large conical cavity divided into three compartments.
or: The thorax is a large conical cavity consisting of three compartments.

Write similar sentences based on the following information:

a) dermis/connective tissue/many blood vessels
b) epidermis/layer of epithelial tissue/dead and growing cells
c) mediastinum/thoracic cavity/pericardium
d) vitreous humor/jelly-like substance/posterior chamber of the eye
e) eye/spherical organ/fatty tissue
f) small intestine/organ of digestion/duodenum, jejunum, ileum

Section 3 Reading

9. As you read this passage, look for the answer to this question:

What are mucous membranes, serous membranes and fibrous membranes composed of?

Membranes

A membrane is a sheet of tissue which covers or lines a surface, or divides an organ into lobes. There are two types of membrane, epithelial and fibrous. Epithelial membranes include mucous membranes and serous membranes.

5 Mucous membranes consist of epithelial tissue with underlying connective tissue called the *lamina propria*. These membranes are wet and slippery, and are found lining the various tracts of the body which open on to the body surface.

Serous membranes are thin, transparent membranes that line closed cavities of the body. They consist of two walls, the parietal layer and the visceral layer, with a potential cavity between the walls which contains some fluid. Each wall

10 consists of a thin layer of either loose connective tissue or fibroelastic tissue, covered with a layer of mesothelium (a kind of epithelium). Nerves and blood and lymph vessels are abundant in serous membranes.

Fibrous membranes are composed of connective tissue only. The *superficial fascia* (subcutaneous tissue), for example, is a combination of loose connective

15 tissue and adipose tissue. It forms a continuous sheet under the skin of the entire body and is firmly attached to the dermis of the skin and to deeper tissues. *Periosteum* is composed of an outer layer of dense connective tissue containing many blood vessels and a deeper layer adjacent to the bone which it surrounds composed of loose connective tissue containing bundles of collagenous fibres

20 and a network of thin elastic fibres.

Now answer these questions:

a) Draw a classification diagram of membranes.
b) What is an organ divided into lobes by?
c) What kind of tissue makes up the deeper layer of mucous membranes and what is its name?
d) What are open body tracts lined with?
e) What is the outer layer of serous membrane walls covered by?
f) What is the layer of tissue superficial to the superficial fascia called?
g) What does superficial fascia lie between?
h) What does the inner layer of periosteum consist of?
i) What does periosteum surround?
j) What are the differences in the composition of superficial fascia and periosteum?

Label these two diagrams:

bundles
a network

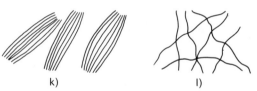

k)   l)

10. Make eight correct sentences from this table by putting the middle parts in the correct order:

a) A sheet of tissue	attached to the dermis	is called a membrane.
b) The lamina propria	containing some fluid	consists of connective tissue.
c) Membranes	covering a surface	are wet and slippery.
d) Membranes	lining closed cavities	are called serous membranes.
e) Connective or fibroelastic tissue	made up *only* of connective tissue	makes up the walls of serous membranes.
f) A potential cavity	lying under the epithelial tissue	lies between the two layers of a serous membrane.
g) Membranes	covered with mesothelium	are called fibrous membranes.
h) The membrane	lining open tracts	is called the superficial fascia.

11. Now indicate what membrane the following consists of:

	mucous membrane	serous membrane	fibrous membrane
a) the lining of the stomach			
b) the pericardium			
c) the pleura			
d) the lining of the mouth			
e) the deep fascia			
f) the sclera			
g) the peritoneum*			
h) the lining of the trachea			

*see glossary

Section 4   Listening

12. Listen to the passage and label the diagram with these words:

nucleus	nucleolus	lipid layer	endoplasmic reticulum
cytoplasm	chromatin	lysosome	Golgi apparatus
cell membrane	protein layer	mitochondrion	

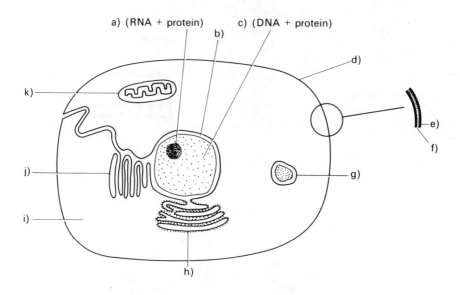

Now complete this description:

> A typical cell consists of a ......, ..., and a ...... The nucleus ...... a single or double ......, consisting of ......, and chromatin, which ...... The cytoplasm ...... various organelles, including ......, ..., ..., ..., etc. The cell membrane ...... The outer and inner layers ...... and the ....

Unit A Revision

1. Look at the diagrams and answer the questions:

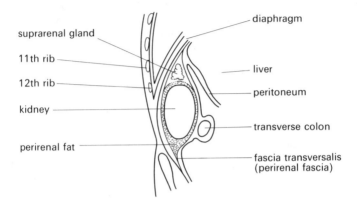

Longitudinal section through the kidney

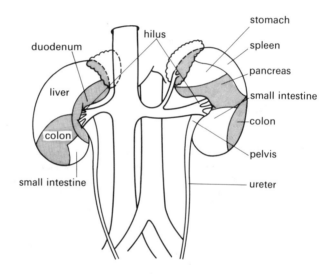

Diagram indicating the principal anterior
and medial relations of the kidneys.
Shaded areas are not covered by peritoneum

  a) Which kidney is higher? Can you guess why?
  b) What is the kidney surrounded by?
  c) What is the name of the concave part of each kidney?
  d) What is the hilus of the right kidney covered by?
  e) What lies between the kidneys?
  f) What separates the kidney superiorly from the suprarenal gland?
  g) What is the shape and position of the right suprarenal gland?
  h) What shape would a transverse section of a kidney be?
  i) What is the shape of the sagittal section in the diagram?
  j) What is the perirenal fascia lined by?

2. Say whether these statements are true or false. Correct the false statements.

a) The kidneys lie on the posterior abdominal wall.
b) The lower pole of the right kidney is covered by the right colic flexure medially and the jejunum laterally.
c) The lower pole of the right kidney is separated anterolaterally from the splenic flexure of the colon by peritoneum.
d) Most of the top part of the right kidney is covered by the diaphragmatic surface of the liver.
e) The pelvis of the ureter is the dilated upper end.
f) The kidneys lie below the ribs.

3. Read the passage and label the diagram using the following words:

major calyx	cortex	pyramid	renal pelvis
minor calyx	medulla	papilla	renal column
capsule	hilus	renal fat	

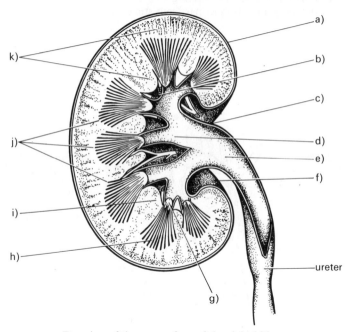

Drawing of the cut surface of the right kidney

The kidney is covered by a thin fibrous sheath, or capsule. The renal blood vessels and the renal pelvis all enter the kidney at the hilus. The renal pelvis divides into three or four major calyces, each of which is divided into several minor calyces. The calyces and renal vessels are embedded in fat.

5   When cut longitudinally, the main part of the kidney is seen to consist of an outer cortex containing the glomeruli (see p. 34) and an inner medulla made up of pyramids. The narrowed ends of these pyramids, the papillae, project into the minor calyces. The medullary pyramids, consisting mainly of collecting ducts, are separated from each other by the renal columns, which are extensions of the
10   cortex and through which the renal vessels pass.

Now answer these questions:

    l) What covers the kidney?
    m) What does the renal fat surround?
    n) What does the perirenal fat surround?
    o) What does the cortex contain?
    p) What is the medulla composed of?
    q) What do the renal columns consist of?
    r) What lies between the calyces and the cortex?

4. Write descriptions of these parts of the kidney using the information given:

Example: cortex/outer part/consisting

The cortex is the outer part of the kidney consisting of glomeruli.

    a) medulla/inner part/composed
    b) papillae/ends of/opening into
    c) renal columns/parts of/lying between
    d) capsule/thin membrane/covering
    e) medullary pyramids/inner part/consisting

5. Look at this:

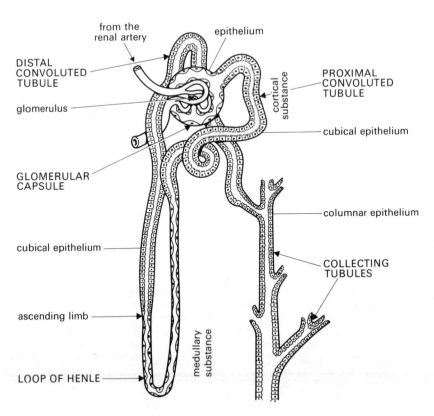

Complete these sentences with suitable names from the diagram:

    a) The working unit of the kidneys is the nephron, which consists of ....
    b) ...... is the cup-shaped end surrounding the glomerulus.
    c) ...... is made up of very thin capillary branches of the renal artery.
    d) ...... consists of two parts: a coiled part which lies near its own glomerulus and a straight section which passes into the descending limb of the loop of Henle.
    e) ...... is the U-shaped section of the tubule, lined by simple squamous epithelium.
    f) The ascending limb, which becomes the ......, coils around the glomerular capsule and then joins one of the ....
    g) ...... pass through the medulla and open on to the surface of the renal papillae into the minor calyces.
    h) ...... are lined by columnar epithelium.
    i) ...... lines the proximal and distal tubules.
    j) ...... is lined by thin, specialised epithelium.

Now join the sentences to make a paragraph about the nephron:

    (Use words like *and, but, which, this,* etc. and *-ing* forms)

Unit 4   Measurement 1

Section 1   Presentation

1. Look at these examples:

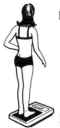

Body weight *is measured in* kilograms (kg).

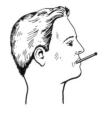

Body temperature *is measured in* degrees Centigrade (°C).

Now make five sentences from this table:

		litres (l).
Blood pressure The quantity of blood in the body Blood haemoglobin content Blood red cell content Blood flow	is measured in	litres (l). litres per minute (l/min). millimetres of mercury (mm/Hg). grams per hundred millilitres (g/100 ml). millions per cubic millimetre (....../cu. mm).

Look at this example:

Q. What is blood pressure measured in?
A. Blood pressure is measured in millimetres of mercury (mm/Hg).

Ask and answer questions about the following, using the information below:

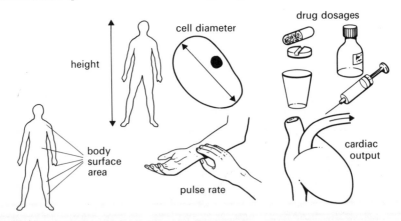

(m) metre	(m²) metre squared ⎱	(l) litre
(cm) centimetre	(sq.m) square metre ⎰	(ml) millilitre
(μm) micron (micrometre)	(g) gram	(cc) cubic centimetre
(l/min) litres per minute	(mg) milligram	(b.p.m.) beats per minute

2. Read this:

(adult pulse c.70 b.p.m.)
The normal pulse rate for a resting adult is about 70 b.p.m.
(oral temperature 36°–37·2°C) (97°–99°F)

Normal temperature in the mouth *ranges* $\left\{{from \atop between}\right\}$ 36° $\left\{{to \atop and}\right\}$ 37·2°C.

Make similar sentences using this information:

a) child's pulse c.90
b) infant's pulse c.120
c) blood pressure (in a young man) 120/80 mm/Hg
d) systolic blood pressure 100–140 mm/Hg.
e) diastolic blood pressure 65–85 mm/Hg.
f) rectal temperature 36·3°–37·6°C
g) axillary temperature 35·5°–36·7°C

3. Look at this table and the example below:

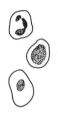

Leucocytes	Normal values		
	average	minimum	maximum
Total number per cu.mm.	7,000	5,000	10,000
Neutrophils	4,300	3,150	6,200
Lymphocytes	2,100	1,500	3,000
Monocytes	375	285	500

The normal leucocyte count for a male ranges from 5,000/cu.mm. to 10,000/cu.mm. with an *average* of 7,000/cu.mm.

Now answer the questions:

a) What is the normal range of values for lymphocytes?
b) What is the average lymphocyte count?
c) What is the normal range of values for monocytes?
d) What is the average monocyte count?
e) Write a sentence about the normal neutrophil count.

4. Look and read:

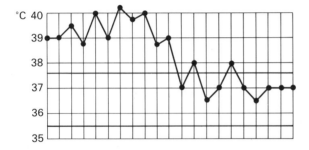

If a patient's temperature is 38°C, it is *above normal*.
If a patient's temperature is 40°C, he has a *high* temperature.
If a patient has a blood pressure of 160/100 mm/Hg, he has a *high* b.p.
If a resting adult's pulse is 100 b.p.m., it is *fast*.

Now comment on these recordings:

a) 36·3°C
b) 85/50 mm/Hg
c) 50 b.p.m. (adult)
d) 140/90 mm/Hg

e) 104°F
f) 125 b.p.m. (infant)
g) 200/120 mm/Hg

h) 34·5°C
i) 115/75 mm/Hg
j) 35·5°C

5. Look at these diagrams:

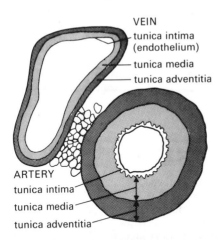

Cross-section of an average sized artery and its accompanying vein (× 80)

Portion of a cross section of the oesophagus (× 20)

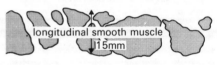

38

Read this:

The section of the oesophagus has been magnified $\begin{cases} \text{by 20.} \\ \text{20 times.} \end{cases}$

In the diagram, *the maximum thickness* of epithelium is 15 mm.
Therefore the *actual* maximum thickness of the epithelium is 0·75 mm. (15/20).

Complete this:

In the diagram, the *minimum* thickness of epithelium is ...... mm.
Therefore ....
The range of thickness of the epithelium is ...... to ...... mm.
The average thickness of the epithelium is ...... mm.

Ask and answer questions from this table:

What is the	average range of	thickness diameter width height etc.	of the	layer of epithelium? submucosal layer? layer of striated muscle? longitudinal muscle layer? artery? vein? arterial tunica adventitia? venous tunica media? etc.

Note: these diagrams may help you:

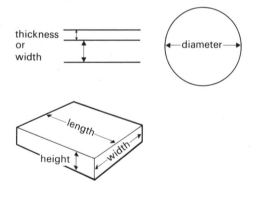

Section 2 Development

6. Look and read:

Incidence of cancer in England

Distribution of systems as % of all sites by sex

This histogram, or bar diagram, shows the number of cancers which occurred in different sites in men and women in England as a percentage of the total number of cases.

The *horizontal axis* represents the percentage of all cases in each sex. The bars along the *vertical axis* represent the different sites of cancer.

From the diagram we can see that:

Cancers of the alimentary tract $\left\{ \begin{matrix} amounted\ to \\ accounted\ for \end{matrix} \right\}$ 26·5 % of all cancers in females.

26·5 % of all cancers in females $\left\{ \begin{matrix} occurred \\ were \end{matrix} \right\}$ in the alimentary tract.

Now answer these questions:

    a) Which type of cancer accounted for 8·5 % of all male cases?
    b) Which site was affected in 4·6 % of all female cases?
    c) Which type of cancer occurred in 28·8 % of all male cases?
    d) Which two types of cancer accounted for over half the total for each sex?

What can you say about:

    e) cancers of the breast in females?
    f) cancers of the urinary system in males?
    g) cancers of the genital system in females?
    h) cancers of the respiratory system in males?
    i) skin cancers in both sexes?

Ask and answer similar questions.

Look at this example:

The incidence of genital cancer was { *higher* in females *than* in males. / *lower* in males *than* in females. }

Now compare the incidence, in males and females, of:

> j) cancers of the buccal cavity and pharynx.
> k) cancers of the urinary system.
> l) lymphoid cancers.

Now look at this example:
> The *highest* incidence of cancer in males was in the respiratory system.

Make sentences about the following in the same way:

> m) ...... lowest ...... males
> n) ...... highest ...... females
> o) ...... lowest ...... females

7. Read this description and then copy the diagram below and add labels:

> This histogram shows an analysis of body composition in five cadavers.
> The vertical axis represents percentage of body weight.
> The bars along the horizontal axis represent (from highest to lowest) water, fat, protein and ash.
> The heights of individual bars are the mean for the five patients.
> The vertical line represents the range.

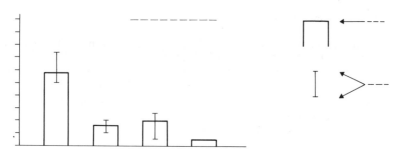

Complete the following sentences:

> a) The amount of water in the human body averages about ...... and ranges ....
>
> b) Protein represents approximately ...... but may vary ....
> c) The maximum value for fat is ....
> d) The minimum recorded amount of water ....
> e) The average value for ash ....

8. Look at this graph and complete the description beside it:

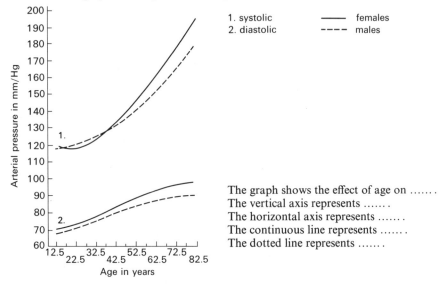

1. systolic   ——— females
2. diastolic   ‒‒‒‒ males

The graph shows the effect of age on ....
The vertical axis represents ....
The horizontal axis represents ....
The continuous line represents ....
The dotted line represents ....

Blood pressure and age

a) What is the average systolic b.p. for males in the age group 20–24?
b) What is the average diastolic b.p. for females in the 30–34 age group?

Ask and answer similar questions.

Between the ages 25–29 and 35–39, the average systolic b.p. in males *increases* from about 120 to approximately 126 mm/Hg.
Between the 10–14 and the 20–24 age groups, the average systolic b.p. in females *decreases* from about 119 to about 117 mm/Hg.

c) What happens to systolic b.p. in females between the 40–44 age group and the 60–64 age group?
d) What happens to their diastolic b.p.?

Ask and answer similar questions.

Read these conclusions which we can draw from the graph:

The graph shows that blood pressure increases with age in both sexes.

Systolic b.p. increases $\left\{\begin{array}{l}\textit{more rapidly} \\ \textit{at a faster rate}\end{array}\right\}$ than diastolic b.p.

The increase in systolic b.p. is $\left\{\begin{array}{l}\textit{more rapid} \\ \textit{faster}\end{array}\right\}$ than the increase in diastolic b.p.

Now compare (in the same way):

e) diastolic b.p. in males and females
f) systolic b.p. in males and females
g) diastolic b.p. in males and females in the age range 10–29
h) systolic and diastolic b.p. in females from 10–34
i) systolic b.p. in males and females in the age range 65–84

9. Draw the axes below and plot the following data on them. Then label the completed graph and give it a title:

Left ventricular volumes with respect to time within the cardiac cycle			
0·0 sec.	170 ml.	0·4 sec.	68 ml.
0·05	175	0·5	90
0·1	172	0·6	117
0·2	130	0·7	136
0·3	86	0·8	159

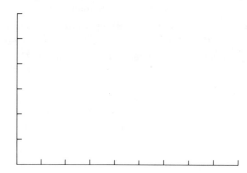

Ask and answer questions using these words/phrases:

a) vertical axis
b) horizontal axis
c) maximum
d) minimum

e) between 0·05 and 0·4 sec.
f) between 0·4 and 0·8 sec.
g) rate of increase/rate of decrease
   (comparison)

Now complete this description of the above graph:

The graph shows the ...... of ...... in the ...... between heart beats. The ...... represents the volume of ...... in ......, and the .... From the graph we can see that the ...... volume occurs at 0·05 ...... when the value is .... From that point the volume ...... until it reaches its ...... of ...... after .... Then it increases to .... Therefore the volume decreases ...... than it increases.

Section 3   Reading

10. Read this passage quickly and choose the best title for it:

Average heart rate
Heart rates in man
Age and heart rate

The average heart rate in man at rest is about 70 beats per minute, although there is a wide variation among individuals, who may have normal rates considerably lower or higher than this. Trained athletes may have a normal rate as low as 50 beats per minute at rest. Their stroke volume, however, is large. Age has an
5 effect on heart rate in that the rate in humans decreases progressively from

approximately 140 beats per minute in the foetus to 120 in the infant, 90 in the child, and 70 in the adult. The heart rate is faster after meals, exercise and emotional excitement.

Choose the correct word or phrase to complete these sentences:

a) ...... states the main idea of the passage.
   A. The first part of the first sentence
   B. The whole of the first sentence
   C. The fourth sentence

b) The second sentence contains ......
   A. a new idea in the passage.
   B. an example of a normal rate higher than average.
   C. an example of a normal rate lower than average.

c) The third sentence explains why 50 b.p.m. for a trained athlete is ......
   A. low.   B. normal.   C. high.   D. restful.

d) The range of normal for resting pulse is approximately ......
   A. 65–75.   B. 60–80.   C. 50–90.   D. 30–110.

e) 'Stroke volume' means ......
   A. a low pulse rate.
   B. the amount of blood pumped out of the heart per beat.
   C. the amount of blood pumped out of the heart per minute.

f) The heart rate is faster after meals because ...... blood than usual is needed by the stomach and intestines.
   A. more   B. less   C. no more

g) Mr X has a pulse of 70 b.p.m. and a stroke volume of 75 ml.
   Mr Y has a pulse of 50 b.p.m. and a stroke volume of 105 ml.
   Therefore Y's heart pumps ....
   A. more blood per beat and more per minute.
   B. more blood per beat but less per minute.
   C. more blood per beat but the same per minute.
   D. less blood per beat and less per minute.

h) Four 25 year old men go to see their doctor. He is quite happy with A who has a pulse of 65 and B whose pulse is 85, but is worried about C, with 53 and D, with 72. Discuss possible explanations for each case.

11. Read this passage to find the answers to these questions:

a) What is 'cardiac index'?
b) What is the range of cardiac index?

The term cardiac index is used to refer to the cardiac output per square metre of body surface area. It is frequently convenient to express the output of the heart per beat as stroke volume, or the cardiac index per beat as stroke index. The resting cardiac index in normal man is approximately 3·3 litres per min per m^2, with a low value of about 2·8 litres per min per m^2. The upper limit of normal is difficult to define because anxiety increases the cardiac output. Cardiac index decreases with age at the rate of approximately 25 ml per min per m^2 per year after early adulthood. Assuming a resting heart rate of 70 beats per min, the normal stroke index is 47 ml per beat for an adult of average size.

Read the passage again and answer these questions:

    c) Here is a summary of the six sentences of the passage.
        Put them in the correct order. (**Note:** one of them refers to *two* sentences.)
        A. Normal values for cardiac index.
        B. Normal value for stroke index.
        C. Definition of cardiac index.
        D. Effect of age on the output of the heart.
        E. Ways of measuring the output of the heart *per beat*.

    d) Rewrite each part of the second sentence to make a sentence similar to the
        first sentence.
        (i)   The term cardiac index is used to refer to the cardiac output per square
              metre of body surface area.

              i.e. C.I. $= \dfrac{\text{C.O.}}{\text{m}^2}$

        (ii) The term stroke volume ....
        (iii) The term ....

    e) Make three sentences from this table:

Cardiac index Stroke volume Stroke index	is calculated by dividing	the cardiac output the cardiac index	by	body surface area in m². pulse rate.

    f) Taking 1·7 m² as the normal body surface area, calculate the normal value for
       cardiac output in a resting man.

    g) Using the information from (f) and taking 70 b.p.m. as normal, calculate the
       stroke volume for a normal adult.

    h) Assuming a resting heart rate of 66 b.p.m., calculate the normal stroke index
       for an average size adult.

Section 4   Listening

12. Look at the graph below and the terms written beside it. Then listen to the passage and label the graph:

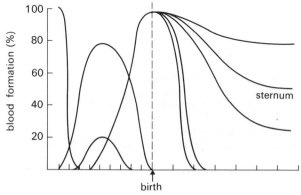

Haematopoiesis in foetal and adult life

Now, describe the graph and say what it tells us about haematopoiesis.

Unit 5   Process 1 Function

Section 1   Presentation

1. Look and read:

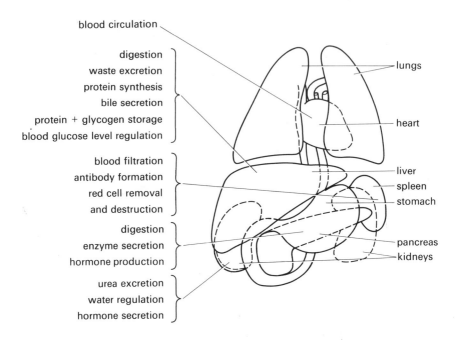

The main organs of the upper abdomen and thorax

Complete these sentences:

a) ...... circulates the blood through the arteries to the tissues.
b) One function of ...... is to regulate the amount of water in the body.
c) ...... is involved in the excretion of a number of waste products.
d) ...... filters the blood.
e) ...... play an important part in the excretion of urea.
f) ...... synthesises proteins from amino acids.
g) One function of ...... is to secrete enzymes.
h) ...... helps to remove and destroy faulty red blood cells.
i) ...... is concerned with storing proteins and glycogen.
j) ...... is involved in digestion as well as producing hormones.
k) ...... functions as an organ of both digestion and excretion.
l) ...... plays a part in forming antibodies.
m) ...... is concerned in the regulation of the level of glucose in the blood.

2. Look at these different ways of expressing function:

The liver *synthesises* proteins.
One function of the liver *is to synthesise* proteins
The liver *functions as* an organ of excretion.

$$\text{The liver}\begin{cases}is\ involved\ in\\is\ concerned\ in\\plays\ a\ part\ in\end{cases}\begin{cases}\text{the excretion of wastes.}\\\text{waste excretion.}\\\text{excreting wastes.}\end{cases}$$

The liver *helps to* excrete wastes.

Complete these sentences, using suitable patterns:

   a) The pancreas ...... hormones.
   b) ...... the liver is to store ....
   c) The spleen ...... blood filtration.
   d) The liver ...... bile.
   e) The kidneys ...... regulating ....
   f) The kidneys also ...... hormones.
   g) The liver helps ...... blood sugar level.
   h) The function of the heart is ....
   i) The pancreas ...... an organ of secretion as well as ....
   j) The liver plays a part ....

Now say each of these sentences a different way.

3. Complete this table:

circulate	circulation	digest	
regulate			formation
	excretion	filter	
secrete			removal
	production	store	
destroy			synthesis

Make six sentences from this table:

Blood circulation The regulation of the amount of water in the body Waste excretion Water regulation The excretion of waste products The circulation of blood to the tissues	is a/the* function of	the liver. the heart. the kidneys.

   * Use 'the' if it is the only function.

In the same way, make two sentences from each of (d) to (m) in exercise 1.

4. Look and read:

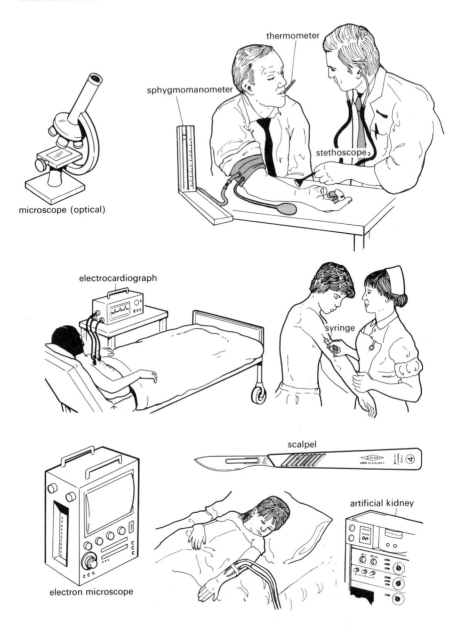

microscope (optical)

sphygmomanometer

thermometer

stethoscope

electrocardiograph

syringe

scalpel

artificial kidney

electron microscope

A microscope is an instrument *which is used for* magnify*ing* objects.
A microscope is an instrument *used for* magnify*ing* objects.
A microscope is an instrument *for* magnify*ing* objects.

Note: An electron microscope is a *machine* for magnifying objects.
It is referred to as a machine because it does or produces something, the reflection of which is then recorded or measured.
('Device' is a general word which can be used in nearly all cases.)

Match these descriptions of function with the diagrams, and include each one in a full sentence like the examples:

a) ...... for measuring temperature.
b) ...... used by doctors for examining the sounds in the chest or other parts of the body.
c) ...... which is used for injecting liquids into the body.
d) ...... for recording electrical changes in heart muscle.
e) ...... used with a stethoscope for measuring blood pressure.
f) ...... like a small light knife used for cutting or incising the body.
g) ...... which is used in cases of severe renal failure for removing waste products from the patient's blood.

Describe some instruments or machines which you use in your practical classes.

Section 2   Development

5. Read the short passages which follow and find the words or phrases which express the functions of the various organs:

(A)

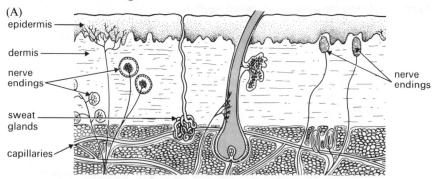

The skin performs many important functions. It serves as a physical barrier, protecting the underlying tissues from injury and harmful bacteria. It contains nerve endings which send information to the brain concerning touch, pain and temperature. It is exceedingly important in the regulation of temperature. It
5 performs some functions as an excretory organ, in that it excretes water, sodium chloride and some urea through its sweat glands. And finally it can function as a means of identification through fingerprints.

Complete this table:

Organ	Function		
Skin	(i)	(ii)	(iii)
Nerve endings	(i)		

Look at the diagram again. Describe each part labelled in the diagram in terms of shape, property, structure, location and function. (Not necessarily all at once.)

Example: Nerve endings have a number of different shapes. They are situated in the bottom layer of the epidermis or just below it, and they send information to the brain concerning touch, pain and temperature.

(B)   The blood transports oxygen from the lungs to the tissues and carbon dioxide from the tissues to the lungs. It carries food materials from the intestines to all parts of the body and returns wastes to the kidneys to be excreted. The blood aids in the regulation of body temperature by distributing the heat produced in
5 active muscles. It plays a vital part in the maintenance of water and salt balance. It is concerned with immunity to disease and protection of the body against invading bacteria.

Say whether these statements are true or false. Correct the false statements.

    a) The blood functions as a carrier of oxygen and carbon dioxide.
    b) The blood is involved in distributing food to the intestines.
    c) Body temperature helps to regulate the blood.
    d) Active muscles help in the production of heat.
    e) The function of the blood is to keep a balance between water and salt.
    f) The blood aids invading bacteria.

Can you think of any more functions of the blood?

6. Read these examples and say which parts describe structure, property, location and function. Note how the sentences are joined together:

Phagocytes are colourless cells found in the tissues as well as the blood.
Phagocytes have the capacity to ingest and destroy foreign particles such as invading bacteria.

→ Phagocytes are colourless cells found in the tissues as well as the blood which have the capacity to ingest and destroy foreign particles such as invading bacteria.

An antibody is a protein formed by the body in response to the presence of an antigen.
Antibodies combine with their antigens and inactivate them.

→ Antibodies, which are proteins formed by the body in response to the presence of antigens, combine with the antigens and inactivate them.

Read the sentences below and label these diagrams:

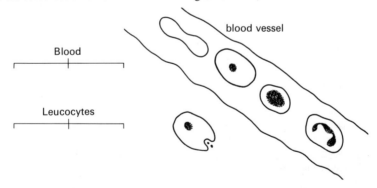

Again say which parts of the sentences describe structure, function, etc.

    a) Granulocytes are capable of engulfing and destroying invading bacteria.
    b) *Plasma* conducts raw materials, such as water, oxygen, glucose, etc., to the tissues and removes waste products.

c) *Haemoglobin* transports oxygen from the lungs to the tissues.

d) The white cells, or leucocytes, include several types: granulocytes, lympho-cytes and monocytes.

e) Lymphocytes are smallish cells with large nuclei.

f) Blood consists of three main components – plasma, erythrocytes and leuco-cytes – each with its own function.

g) *Granulocytes are* also known as polymorphonuclear leucocytes because of their segmented nuclei.

h) *Monocytes are* phagocytic.

i) Plasma is a pale yellow, clear fluid.

j) Normal erythrocytes (red cells) are circular, biconcave discs without nuclei, containing haemoglobin.

k) *Lymphocytes* are concerned with immunity and form antibodies.

l) Monocytes are large round cells.

Now arrange the sentences to form a paragraph.
Join function sentences to other descriptions, as in the examples, leaving out the words in italics.
Finally, write out the paragraph.

7. Read this:

Medical textbooks describe both well-known functions and functions which are being investigated by current research. These functions may be certain or not so certain.

Example: *Recent research has demonstrated*   } a number of different
           Investigators have provided evidence of }
           types of cell with endocrine function.
           These are *certain*.

      ⌈ Eosinophil leucocytes *probably* leave the tissues through the lymphatics.
      | *It is thought that* eosinophil leucocytes leave the tissues through the lymphatics.
      ⌊ Eosinophil leucocytes *are thought to* leave the tissues through the lymphatics.
       These are *not* certain.

Now expand these sentences to show whether they are certain (C) or uncertain (U):

a) All endothelial cells have phagocytic ability.   (U)

b) The thymus produces a factor which plays a part in making lymphocytes attack antigens.   (C)

c) In the child, the thymus controls the other lymphoid tissues.   (U)

Section 3 Reading

8. Read the passage and label the diagram:

The spleen is a highly vascular, lymphoid organ which functions as part of both the reticuloendothelial system (RES) and the haemopoietic system. It has been evident for many years that clearance from the blood of injured blood cells is a function of the RES, and the most important organ of the RES in this process of
5 filtration is the spleen, which allows normal cells to pass through but can detain and destroy abnormal cells. Investigators have demonstrated, for example, that in the condition known as hereditary spherocytosis the spleen selectively detains the red cells (spherocytes) and destroys them. Other researchers have shown that the spleen traps immature red cells, including many reticulocytes, which prob-
10 ably ripen there and return to the circulation. The spleen and the bone marrow are the two RES organs most involved in this detention of nucleated red cells.

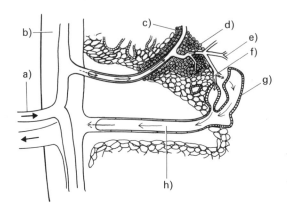

The formation of blood cells is an important function of the spleen in the foetus. In the adult, however, the spleen is only concerned with lymphocyte formation, although it is thought to aid in forming erythrocytes in certain
15 circumstances.

The spleen consists of red pulp and white pulp, covered by a fibroelastic capsule. The white pulp is composed of sheaths of lymphatic tissue (consisting mainly of lymphocytes and macrophages) which surround branches of the splenic artery. In places these sheaths are enlarged to form lymphatic follicles,
20 which are sites of lymphocyte production. The lymphocytes, in turn, play a part in the formation of antibodies. The red pulp, on the other hand, which makes up most of the spleen, is composed of erythrocytes in contact with lymphocytes and reticuloendothelial cells (macrophages), all surrounding numerous vascular sinusoids. The blood from the arterioles probably passes through the red pulp
25 and the filtered blood passes into the sinusoids, which join venules carrying the blood to the splenic vein. Some other people, however, think that blood passes directly from the arterioles into the sinusoids.

9. Give each of the three paragraphs a heading:

    a) The structure of the spleen
    b) The haemopoietic function of the spleen
    c) The filtering function of the spleen

Complete these sentences:

    d) One function of the RES is ....
    e) The bone marrow plays a part ....
    f) The lymph follicles are involved ....
    g) ...... is a function of the lymphocytes.
    h) The function of the red pulp ....
    i) The sinusoids ....
    j) Which sentence or part of a sentence in the passage summarises the main function of the spleen most completely?

10. Answer these questions:

    a) Does the spleen detain all red blood cells in hereditary spherocytosis?
    b) What are spherocytes and why does the spleen detain them? (**Note:** sphero-cyte.)
    c) What is a reticulocyte and why is it detained by the spleen?
    d) List all the examples of abnormal cells mentioned in the passage. Can you think of any others?

Say whether these statements are true, probably true, or false:

    e) The spleen is thought to destroy spherocytes.
    f) There is evidence that immature erythrocytes are detained by the spleen.
    g) Reticulocytes detained in the spleen become mature and then leave the spleen.
    h) It is thought that the bone marrow traps nucleated red cells.
    i) Erythrocyte formation is a function of the spleen.
    j) The red pulp of the spleen plays an important part in the removal of abnormal erythrocytes.

11. Write a summary of the functions of the spleen.

Section 4   Listening

12. Look and read:

The gallbladder:
    a) Discharge of bile into duodenum
    b) Storage and concentration of bile
    c) Digestion of proteins
    d) Secretion of cholestrol
    e) Maintenance of bile pressure

Bile salts:
    f) Activation of digestive enzymes
    g) Stimulation of gallbladder contraction
    h) Activation of pancreatic lipase
    i) Stimulation of fat digestion

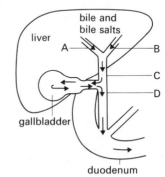

Listen to the passage and label A to D on the diagram.
Listen again and write down the order of those functions which occur in the passage.
Listen a third time and say whether each function is certain or uncertain.

Unit 6 Process 2 Actions in Sequence

Section 1 Presentation

1. Look and read:

FACULTY OF MEDICINE				
1st yr.	2nd yr.	3rd yr.	4th yr.	5th yr.
anatomy		surgery		radiology
histology	physiology	pathology	special pathology	paediatrics
biology / micro-biology	biochemistry	pharmacology	obstetrics & gynaecology	
bacteri-ology / virology / parasit-ology		epidemi-ology	tropical diseases	otolaryngology
genetics			medicine	

Histology comes *before* physiology.
Microbiology is studied *after* biology.
During their study of histology the students also study biology and microbiology.
They study bacteriology $\begin{cases} \text{\textit{at the same time as} microbiology.} \\ \text{\textit{as} they study microbiology.} \end{cases}$
They study biology and microbiology *while* they study histology (and anatomy).
They begin the study of physiology *when* they enter the second year.
Radiology is not studied *until* they enter the fifth year.
Surgery is studied from the beginning of the third *until* the end of the fourth year.

Now answer these questions:

   a) What subjects do they study before epidemiology?
   b) What do they study after physiology and before obstetrics and gynaecology?
   c) What subjects are studied only until the middle of the first year?
   d) Which subject is not studied until the middle of the second year?
   e) What else do they study while they study otolaryngology?
   f) What is studied at the same time as genetics?
   g) How many subjects do they study in their second year?
   h) Which seven subjects do they also study during their study of obstetrics and
      gynaecology?
   i) What happens when they reach the middle of the second year?
   j) What else do they study as they study pharmacology and surgery?

Now write statements about your own programme, using the words

     before, after, during, at the same time as, as, while, when, until

2. Look and read:

Development of the human embryo

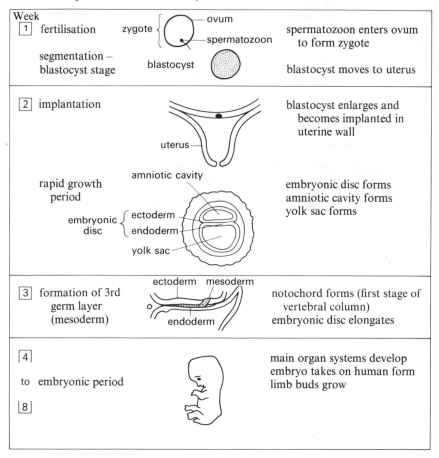

Week			
1	fertilisation	zygote {— ovum / — spermatozoon	spermatozoon enters ovum to form zygote
	segmentation – blastocyst stage	blastocyst	blastocyst moves to uterus
2	implantation	uterus	blastocyst enlarges and becomes implanted in uterine wall
	rapid growth period	amniotic cavity / embryonic disc { ectoderm / endoderm / yolk sac	embryonic disc forms / amniotic cavity forms / yolk sac forms
3	formation of 3rd germ layer (mesoderm)	ectoderm mesoderm / endoderm	notochord forms (first stage of vertebral column) / embryonic disc elongates
4 to 8	embryonic period		main organ systems develop / embryo takes on human form / limb buds grow

(*Preceding actions*)

The embryo segments { *before* it *is* implanted. / *before* be*ing* implanted.* / *before* implant*ation*.

Prior to the implant*ation* of the embryo, there is the segmentation stage.

Complete these:

      a) The mesoderm forms before ....
      b) Before the embryonic disc forms, ...
      c) The ectoderm and the endoderm form ....
      d) Prior to ...... the blastocyst becomes implanted in the uterine wall.
      e) Before entering the rapid growth period, ...

(* **Note:** the subject of the first part must be the same as the subject of the 2nd part.)

(*Simultaneous actions*)

As⎫
While⎭ the zygote *segments*, it moves to the uterus.

During ⎰segment*ation*⎱ the zygote moves to the uterus.
⎱the segmentation *stage*⎰

Complete these:

f) As the mesoderm begins to form ....
g) ...... the yolk sac forms.
h) The limb buds grow while ....
i) During the third week ....
j) During the embryonic period ....

(*Following actions*)

When ⎰the ovum is fertilised, the zygote is formed.
⎱it is fertilised, the ovum becomes the zygote.

After⎫ the blastocyst is implanted, there is a period of rapid growth.
When⎭

After ⎰*be*ing implanted⎱ the blastocyst grows rapidly.*
⎱implant*ation*   ⎰

(* See note on page 55.)

Complete these:

k) When ......, it grows rapidly.
l) ......, the limb buds begin to form.
m) After ...... the yolk sac, ...
n) After forming in the second week, ... in the third week.
o) On reaching the uterus ....

(*Completed actions*)

By the beginning of the embryonic period, the three germ layers have formed.
By the end of the embryonic period, the embryo has taken on human form.

Complete these:

p) By the end of the second week ....
q) ...... the zygote has segmented.
r) By the third week ....

The embryonic period continues *until* the end of the 8th week.

⎧the third week.
The mesoderm does not form *until* ⎨the ectoderm and endoderm have begun to
⎩   form.

s) The blastocyst continues moving until ....
t) The embryonic disc does not form until ....
u) The main organs do not begin to develop ....
v) The ovum cannot segment until ....

Section 2   Development

3. Read this:

Schistosomiasis is a disease found all over the world. It is spread by a small
fluke, or flatworm, which acts as a parasite during one stage of its life cycle to
water-snails, and during another to man. Three species cause human disease:
Schistosoma haematobium is found in parts of Africa, in parts of Spain and the
5 Middle East; *S. mansoni* in Africa and South America; *S. japonicum* in the Far
East.

Look and read:

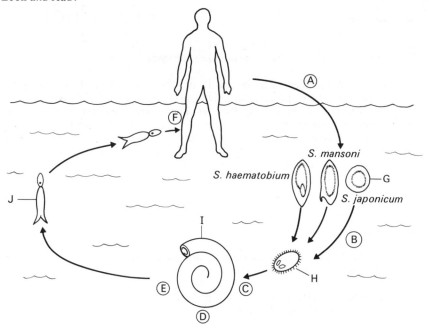

Schistosomiasis: 1st stage of fluke's life cycle

In these areas, flukes' eggs are present in slow-moving water. When the eggs
hatch, the embryos invade the bodies of the water-snails which act as host
during this first stage of the fluke's life cycle. The embryos grow and return to
the water when they have developed into cercariae. Then they swim freely until
they are able to penetrate the skin of other humans and enter their circulation.

Now match labels (a) to (d) with G to J, and (e) to (j) with A to F in the diagram:

a) cercaria	e) cercariae return to water	h) eggs hatch
b) eggs	f) embryos invade snails	i) eggs excreted
c) embryo	g) cercariae penetrate human	j) embryos grow into
d) snail	skin	cercariae

57

4. Look at this diagram and choose the correct words to complete the passage below:

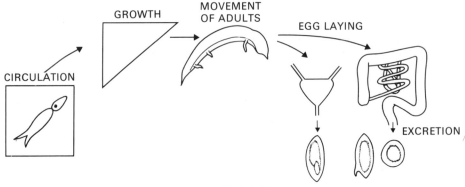

2nd stage of fluke's life cycle

(Before/When) they enter the circulation, the second stage of the fluke's life cycle begins. First the (cercariae/adult worms) pass through the system (while/ until) they reach the veins of the liver. There they remain for some time and during this stage they grow into (cercariae/adult worms). Then the (cercariae/ adult worms) move to the urinary bladder – in the case of *S. haematobium*, or the intestines – *S. mansoni*, *S. japonicum*. Next the adults (are excreted/lay their eggs). Finally the eggs are excreted in the urine or faeces, but (before/after) leaving the body the eggs cause inflammation in the affected organ. (On/While) being excreted into water containing snails, the eggs can begin the life cycle again.

Complete these sentences:

    a) The flukes begin the 2nd stage of their life cycle on ....
    b) While the fluke is in the liver ....
    c) Before reaching the veins of the liver ....
    d) After ......, the adults lay their eggs.
    e) Inflammation occurs during ....

Complete this brief summary of the 2nd stage:

    First ......, where they grow into ....
    Then .... Next .... Finally ....

5. Look at this:

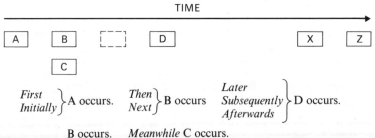

Now look at this diagram of what happens in the body after invasion by cercariae:
STAGE:

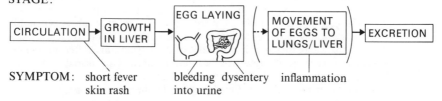

CIRCULATION → GROWTH IN LIVER → EGG LAYING → MOVEMENT OF EGGS TO LUNGS/LIVER → EXCRETION

SYMPTOM: short fever   bleeding dysentery   inflammation
            skin rash   into urine

Complete this description by matching the sentences on the right with the words on the left:

a) Initially   there are no symptoms for a long time.
b) Afterwards   there is bleeding into the urine or dysentery.
c) Meanwhile   the eggs are excreted and the bleeding and dysentery cease.
d) Then, (A),   there is a short fever and skin rash. (B).
e) Subsequently the cercariae grow in the liver into adults which later move to the bladder or intestines.
f) Finally   the eggs may cause a mild but long-lasting inflammation (C).

Now put the following phrases in place of A, B and C above, and write out the complete paragraph:

g) after being carried to the liver or lungs.
h) when the eggs are laid.
i) These occur while the cercariae are still circulating.

Section 3   Reading

6. Read the passage and put these diagrams in the correct order:

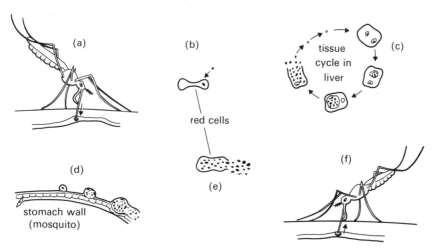

Malaria

Malaria is an infectious disease caused by a minute animal parasite (protozoon) transmitted by mosquitoes, one of the commonest causes of sickness and death in the world. (A) But how does malaria develop?

First the mosquito sucks blood from an infected person. Then the parasites
5   breed in the mosquito's stomach, and after about ten days their offspring invade
the salivary glands. At this stage the mosquito is infectious: when it bites a
human subject it gives an injection of parasites in a droplet of saliva. When this
happens the young parasites are carried in the patient's blood to the liver and
other organs where they multiply without causing symptoms. After this period
10   of incubation (B) parasites return to the blood stream and invade red blood cells.
There they multiply rapidly and rupture the cells, releasing countless parasites
to invade other red cells (C). Finally, when this happens, the patient has an
attack of fever.

    The attack commonly begins with headache and violent shivering (rigor). (D)
15   After anything from an hour to a day the symptoms disappear until the next
batch of parasites is released, with further destruction of red cells. All types of
malaria cause attacks of fever at more or less regular intervals, and increasing
anaemia from loss of blood cells. (E)

Now summarise the development of the disease by copying and completing this flow
diagram. (**Note:** decide first which paragraph you need.)

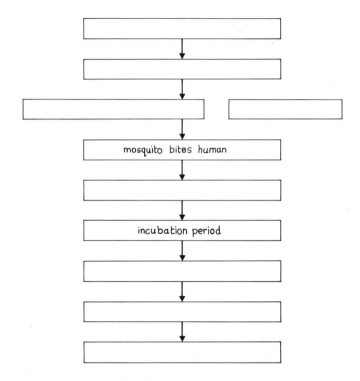

Development of malaria

Now summarise the sequence of events in the attacks of fever:

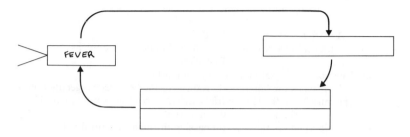

Match the following sentences/clauses with A, B, C, D and E in the text:

    a) This stage – the 'cold stage' – lasts 20 to 60 minutes and is followed by a 'hot stage' of three to eight hours with temperatures of 40° to 42°C.

    b) There are three main species of protozoon known to infect man: *Plasmodium vivax* causes tertian malaria; *P. malaria* causes quartan malaria; and *P. falciparum* causes malignant tertian malaria.

    c) Muscle pains and splenomegaly are also common.

    d) which in turn are destroyed either immediately or by phagocytosis in the liver or the spleen.

    e) which varies from ten to fourteen days in vivax and falciparum malaria to eighteen days to six weeks in quartan infections.

Section 4   Listening

7. Listen to the passage and label this diagram of the heart, using the initial letters of the terms beside the diagram:

Example: IVC = *inferior vena cava*

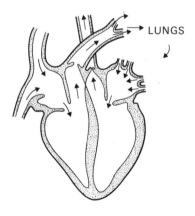

inferior vena cava
superior vena cava
left atrium
right atrium
left ventricle
right ventricle
aortic valve
pulmonary valve
mitral valve
tricuspid valve
pulmonary arteries
pulmonary veins
aorta

Now choose the correct word/phrase to complete these sentences.
Check your answers as you listen to the passage a second time.

    a) ...... passing into the right atrium the blood flows through the tricuspid valve.
        A. After   B. Before

    b) The tricuspid valve closes ...... the pulmonary valve opens.
        A. as   B. before

    c) The blood does not take up oxygen until it ....
        A. reaches the lungs.   B. returns to the heart as oxygenated blood.

    d) The muscles of the left ventricle and ...... contract simultaneously.
        A. left atrium   B. right ventricle

    e) The blood enters the ...... on passing through the mitral valve.
        A. left atrium   B. left ventricle

    f) ...... the ejection of blood into the aorta the aortic valve opens.
        A. Before   B. During

    g) The blood from the superior vena cava enters the heart ...... that from the inferior vena cava.
        A. before   B. at the same time as

    h) The pressure in the right ventricle increases ...... the contraction of the muscles.
        A. after   B. during

    i) The pulmonary valve remains ...... while the blood flows into the ....
        A. closed   B. open   C. pulmonary arteries.   D. pulmonary veins.

    j) The mitral valve does not ...... until the left ventricular muscles contract.
        A. close   B. open

8. Join these pairs of sentences using one of the words in brackets and making any other necessary changes:

    Example: The pulmonary valve remains closed.
                 The pressure in the right ventricle forces the pulmonary valve open.
                                            (until/after)

            → The pulmonary valve remains closed until it is forced open by the pressure in the right ventricle.

    a) Carbon dioxide is not given up by the blood.
        The blood reaches the lungs.   (until/after)

    b) The pressure inside the left ventricle increases.
        The opening of the aortic valve occurs.   (Meanwhile/Prior to)

    c) Pressure forces blood into the aorta.
        Blood flows to the tissues.   (Then/As)

    d) The pulmonary valve opens.
        The blood flows into the pulmonary arteries.   (When/During)

    e) The blood reaches the lungs.
        Oxygen is taken up.   (On/During)

Unit B   Revision

1. Look and answer:

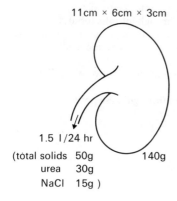

11cm × 6cm × 3cm

1.5 l/24 hr

(total solids 50g
      urea   30g
      NaCl   15g)

140g

a) What is the approximate weight of a normal kidney?
b) What is the length of each kidney?
c) What is the width of each kidney?
d) What is the thickness of each kidney?
e) How much urine is produced per minute?
f) What is the percentage of urea in the solid constituents of urine?

2. Read this:

Glomerular filtration

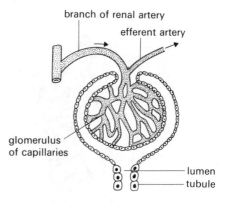

branch of renal artery

efferent artery

glomerulus of capillaries

lumen

tubule

Glomerular capsule

A filter or sieve is a device which separates large and small particles by retaining the larger particles and allowing the smaller particles
5 to pass through. In the kidney it is the glomerulus of each nephron which filters the blood by allowing blood constituents having a molecular weight of less than 68,000 to
10 pass through into the tubules, but retaining any larger molecules and particles in the blood capillaries. Electron microscope studies have shown pores 0·1 μm in diameter between the capillary and the lumen of the tubule which are thought to be associated with this filtering action.

Blood constituents	
Molecular weight above 68,000	Molecular weight below 68,000
Red cells White cells Platelets Plasma proteins	Water Food substances (glucose, amino acids, etc.) Inorganic salts Waste products (urea, uric acid, etc.)

63

Complete these:

     a) ...... is the function of a sieve.
     b) ...... is the function of the glomerulus.
     c) ...... is the function of an electron microscope.

Say whether these statements are true or false. Correct the false statements.

     d) Red cells probably pass through the capillary into the tubules.
     e) Sodium chloride has been shown to pass through into the tubules.
     f) It can be demonstrated that proteins normally pass through the glomerulus.
     g) Plasma proteins have a higher molecular weight than amino acids.
     h) The blood consists of urea and uric acid.
     i) It is thought that the diameter of the holes, or pores, between capillary and
        lumen is $0.1\,\mu m$.
     j) It has been shown that the blood is filtered through these pores.

3. Read this passage and choose a title for it:

     a) The kidney   c) Glomerular filtration
     b) Renal function   d) Tubular reabsorption

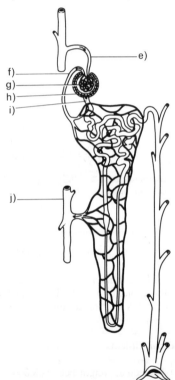

Diagram of nephron

Blood enters the glomerulus by way of an afferent arteriole of the renal artery
and after circulating through it leaves via an efferent arteriole, which leads to a
second capillary network around the tubule. The function of this secondary

network will be discussed later, but the blood does not return to the renal vein
5 until it has passed through this network.

When the blood passes through the glomerulus a certain amount is filtered into the glomerular capsule. This is known as the glomerular filtrate. From the capsule the filtrate makes its way along the lumen of the tubule and while doing this the tubule cells selectively reabsorb the filtrate constituents. Glucose and
10 other food substances, for example, are completely reabsorbed in the proximal tubule. Water is almost completely reabsorbed: of the 125 ml of glomerular filtrate only about 1 ml appears as urine. About three quarters of this water is reabsorbed in the proximal tubule; the rest in the distal tubule and collecting duct (A). Inorganic salts are reabsorbed mainly in the proximal tubules also,
15 but they are also reabsorbed in the next two parts of the nephron. (B). Waste products such as urea are partially reabsorbed in the proximal tubule but much of these is excreted in the urine. Finally, these various reabsorbed substances pass from the tubular cells into the capillary network (C).

(D) certain substances are actively secreted into the lumen by the tubule
20 cells. (E). PAH does not appear in the renal veins at all because it is completely excreted by both filtration in the capsule and tubular secretion in the next part of the nephron.

(F) the remaining filtrate joins the filtrate from thousands of other nephrons before finally emptying into the renal pelvis and the ureter. By this time it has
25 become urine.

Match these labels with (e) to (j) in the diagram:

| afferent arteriole | glomerulus | lumen |
| efferent arteriole | glomerular capsule | renal vein |

4. Match these clauses/sentences with A to F in the passage:

a) Potassium is unusual in that it seems to be completely reabsorbed in the proximal tubule and to be re-excreted in the distal tubule.
b) Such substances include para-aminohippuric acid (PAH) and penicillin.
c) After passing through the nephron,
d) In addition to being filtered by the glomerulus,
e) but not in the loop of Henle which is impermeable to water.
f) before returning via the renal vein to the circulation.

5. Each of the following nephrons represents all the nephrons in the kidneys, and shows in diagrammatic form (and therefore approximately) what happens to different substances in the kidneys. Match these labels with the diagrams:

water   urea   PAH   glucose

a)

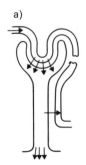

b)

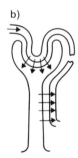

c)

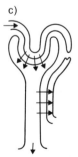

d)

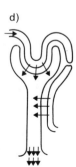

6. Answer these questions:

   a) What is the function of the 'secondary network' (ll. 3 and 4)?
   b) What are the functions of the tubule cells?
   c) Describe what happens to urea in the kidneys.
   d) Describe what happens to potassium in the kidneys.
   e) What happens to substances filtered by the glomerulus but not excreted?
   f) Where does tubular secretion of PAH occur?
   g) What happens prior to the secretion of PAH into the lumen by the tubule cells? (Describe what happens to PAH in the kidneys.)
   h) Describe what takes place in:
      (i) the capsule   (ii) the proximal tubule   (iii) the loop of Henle
      (iv) the distal tubule   (v) the collecting ducts   (vi) the tubule cells

7. Summarise the main points described in the passage using these words:

   Initially ...... Then ...... Meanwhile ...... Subsequently ......
   Eventually ...... Finally ......

Unit 7   Measurement 2 Quantity

Section 1   Presentation

1. Look at this table:

Recommended daily intakes (for Britain)				
	Woman 18–55	Pregnant woman	Lactating woman	Old woman (75+)
Carbohydrate	325 g	350	390	280
Fat	75 g	85	95	65
Protein	55 g	60	68	48
Thiamin	0·9 mg	1·0	1·1	0·7
Ascorbic acid	30 mg	60	60	30
Vitamin A	750 μg	750	1,200	750
Vitamin D	2·5 μg	10	10	2·5
Calcium	500 mg	1,200	1,200	500
Iron	12 mg	15	15	10
Copper	trace	trace	trace	trace

Ask questions from this table and answer them using the information above:

How much		protein		an average woman	
		calcium		a pregnant woman	
	grams	thiamin	does	a pregnant woman	require
How many	milligrams of	vit. A		a lactating woman	daily?
	micrograms	etc.		an old woman	

2. Read this:

A pregnant woman needs $\begin{cases}\text{twice}\\\text{two times}\end{cases}$ as much vit. C as an average woman.

Compare:

    a) pregnant – average (vit. D)
    b) lactating – average (calcium)

A is one third/33% larger than B. (i.e. C = ⅓B)
B is one quarter/25% smaller than A (i.e. C = ¼A)

A pregnant woman needs 25% more iron than an average woman.
An average woman needs 20% less iron than a pregnant woman.

Compare:

c) lactating – average   (protein)   f) old – average   (carbohydrate)
d) pregnant – average   (thiamin)   g) old – average   (thiamin)
e) lactating – pregnant   (vit. A)

Look at this example:

An old woman needs about 12% less of this than an average woman.

What is it?   Answer: iron.

Now ask and answer similar questions.

3. Look and read:

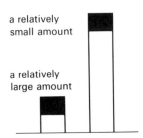

a relatively
small amount

a relatively
large amount

A pregnant woman requires 10 µg vit. D, which is a very small amount indeed, but, compared with the amount required by an average woman, it is a *relatively* large amount.

Compared with an average woman, a pregnant woman needs *much* more vit. D, *considerably* more calcium and vit. C, and *slightly* more carbohydrate, fat and protein.

Complete these:

a) Compared with an average woman, a lactating woman requires much more
   ......, ... vitamin A, and ...... thiamin.
b) Compared with a pregnant woman, a lactating woman needs ....
c) By comparison with an average woman, an old woman needs ....

4. Compare the amounts in this table with the recommended daily intakes in exercise 1:

	Thiamin (mg/100 g)	Vit. C (mg/100 g)	Vit. A (µg/100 g)	Vit. D (per 100 g)
Beef	0·05–0·1	trace	10–20	trace
Milk	0·04–0·06		20–50	trace – 0·2 µg
Eggs	0·1 –0·15	trace	200–400	4–10 µg (yolk)
Wheat (germ)	2·5 –5·6			
Citrus fruits		25–60		
Halibut liver oil			1,000,000– 2,000,000	0·5–10 mg

Beef contains a *significant* amount of thiamin.
The vitamin C content of beef is *negligible*.
Vitamin A is present in *particularly high concentrations* in halibut liver oil.

Now identify these:

a) These contain significant quantities of vitamin C only.
b) These are found in significant amounts in eggs and halibut liver oil.
c) This contains a particularly high concentration of vitamin D.
d) This contains a negligible quantity of vitamin D and a small but significant amount of vitamin A.
e) This is present in significant amounts in eggs and particularly in wheat germ.

Section 2   Development

5. Look and read:

Biochemical aids in diagnosing nutritional deficiency (adult values)

Nutrient	Test*	Level suggesting deficiency	Usual range
Protein	Total protein (S) g/100 ml	<6.0	6·5–8·6
Vitamin A	Vitamin A (P) µg/100 ml	<10.0	20–49
Vitamin E	Tocopherols (P) mg/100 ml	<0.4	0·6–1·5
Vitamin C	Ascorbate (B) mg/100 ml	<0.3	0·4–1·0
Thiamin	Pyruvate (B) mg/100 ml	>1.0	0·3–0·9
Iron	Iron (S) µg/100 ml	<50	60–160
Copper	Copper (S) µg/100 ml	<75	81–147

* P, plasma; S, serum; B, whole blood.

A laboratory finding of 7·9 g/100 ml serum indicates {an *adequate* protein level. / a *sufficient* supply of protein.

A laboratory finding of 0·15 mg ascorbate per 100 ml blood indicates that } there is a {*shortage* / *deficiency* / *lack*} of vit. C.
If the concentration of ascorbate in the blood is less than 0·3 mg/100 ml then } there is *not enough* vitamin C.
the vitamin C level is {*inadequate.* / *insufficient.*}

When the plasma value for vitamin A falls to 10 µg/100 ml, the *deficient* state is probably present.

Now choose the correct word or phrase to complete these sentences:

a) A laboratory finding of 68 µg/100 ml serum indicates that there is ...... copper in the body.   A. a deficiency of   B. an adequate amount of
b) When the plasma value for vitamin A is 19 µg/100 ml there is probably ...... vitamin A.   A. a sufficient quantity of   B. a lack of
c) A laboratory finding of 0·25 mg tocopherol per 100 ml plasma suggests that the vitamin E level is ....   A. adequate   B. inadequate
d) If the serum iron level is between 55 and 75 µg/100 ml then there is probably ...... in the body.   A. enough iron   B. a shortage of iron
e) If the concentration of pyruvate in the blood is more than 1 mg/100 ml then ....
A. the thiamin level is adequate.   B. there is not enough thiamin.

Now comment on these findings:

- f) serum copper level 43 μg/100 ml
- g) blood ascorbate level 0·9 mg/100 ml
- h) plasma tocopherol level 0·9 mg/100 ml
- i) serum protein level 4·9 g/100 ml
- j) serum iron level 43–48 μg/100 ml

6. Look and read:

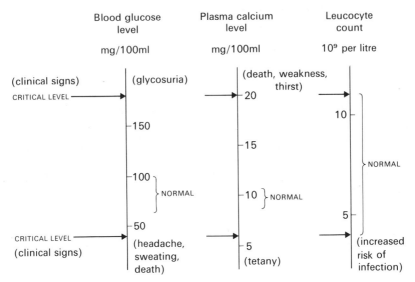

If the plasma calcium *exceeds* 20 mg/100 ml

then there is
$\left\{ \begin{array}{l} \textit{an excess of} \\ \textit{an excessive amount of} \\ \textit{too much} \end{array} \right\}$ calcium

and clinical signs will be evident (e.g. thirst, weakness).
This condition is known as *hyper*calcaemia.

Note: $\left. \begin{array}{l} \textit{too little} \\ \textit{too much} \end{array} \right\}$ calcium, blood, etc. $\left. \begin{array}{l} \textit{too few} \\ \textit{too many} \end{array} \right\}$ cells, tablets, etc.

Write similar sentences, using these notes to help you:

- a) blood glucose >180/......-glycaemia
- b) leucocyte count >11 × 10⁹/leucocytosis
- c) plasma vitamin A >165 μg/100 ml/toxic effects/......-vitaminosis A

Complete these:

- d) Oedema can be defined as ...... water in the tissue fluid; by which we mean that ...... (>normal amount of water).
- e) Polycythaemia is a disease of the blood in which there are too many red cells; i.e. ......
- f) Hyperplasia refers to ...... growth of tissue by multiplication of its cells.
- g) Hypertrophy is ...... tissue growth by enlargement (without multiplication) of ....

7. Complete this sentence, using information from the two previous exercises:

    a) If the plasma calcium level falls below ......, then there is ...... and .... This ...... *hypo*calcaemia.

Write similar sentences about:

    b) blood glucose level
    c) leucocyte count (leucopenia)

Complete these sentences:

    d) Anaemia literally means ...... blood, but in fact ...... haemoglobin or ...... erythrocytes.
    e) Anoxia is a condition in which ...... oxygen; that is to say the supply of oxygen to the tissues ....
    f) An overdose of a drug occurs when a patient takes too much of a particular drug, or ...... tablets; i.e. ....
    g) The pancreatic hormone insulin helps the uptake of glucose from the blood by the tissues. In diabetes mellitus there is a deficiency of insulin, which means that the blood sugar level ...... because glucose is taken up too slowly by the tissues and therefore accumulates in the blood. But in ......-insulinism, or after an overdose of insulin in a diabetic, the blood sugar level is ......-creased.
    h) ......-glycaemia is the main clinical sign of diabetes. Hypoglycaemia, on the other hand, can result from ...... production of insulin.

8. Look at this diagram of a capillary:

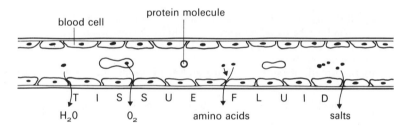

Water molecules are *small enough to* pass through capillary walls.

Protein molecules are $\begin{cases}\textit{not small enough}\\ \textit{too large}\end{cases}$ *to* pass through capillary walls.

Note: small *enough* to = CAN pass through; (reason) – small
                                    so small (in relation to the size of the gap) that they *can* pass through

        too large to   = canNOT pass through; (reason) – large
                                      so large (in relation to the size of the gaps) that they can*not* pass through

Now make similar sentences about:

    a) amino acids b) sugars c) erythrocytes d) salts

    (**Note:** cf. Unit B, exercise 2)

9. Look and read:

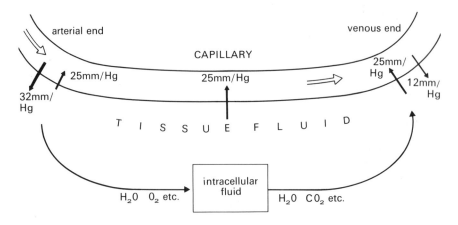

The proteins in the plasma exert an osmotic pressure of 25 mm/Hg.
At the arterial end of the capillaries blood pressure is 32 mm/Hg.

Therefore

    the blood pressure is *high enough to* force water into the tissue fluid.

or:

    The osmotic pressure is $\begin{cases} \textit{not high enough to} \\ \textit{too low to} \end{cases}$ prevent water being forced in-to the tissue fluid.

Choose the correct answer(s):

    a) At the venous end, the pressure has fallen to 12 mm/Hg.
        Therefore the blood pressure is ...... to force more water out.
        A. too high   B. too low   C. not high enough   D. not low enough
    or, in other words:
    b) the osmotic pressure is ...... to draw water back into the blood from the tissue
        fluid.

        A. too high   B. too low   C. high enough   D. low enough

Now complete these sentences:

    c) If the blood pressure falls below a critical level, it is then ...... to force water,
        etc. into the tissue fluid.
    d) In hypocalcaemia there is ...... for proper bone development.
    e) When the blood glucose level exceeds ......, the kidneys cannot ...... all the
        glucose, and some glucose appears ...... (glycosuria); i.e. when the blood
        glucose exceeds a critical level, ... for the kidneys to reabsorb.
    f) In tissue hypoxia, when the tension of the gas is low, the pressure head of
        oxygen in the capillaries ...... to provide distant cells with sufficient oxygen
        for their metabolic needs.
    g) Normal erythrocytes ...... to pass through the filtering mechanism of the
        spleen, whereas abnormal erythrocytes ....
    h) Oedema, or ...... tissue fluid, can occur when the plasma protein falls below a
        critical level with the result that the osmotic pressure is ...... to draw the
        water back into the blood.
    i) Oedema also occurs in cases of high venous blood pressure because then the
        blood pressure at the venous end of ......, with the result that ....

j) Oedema can also be caused by capillary damage, because damaged capillaries are permeable to proteins and therefore ....

Read this:

At the arterial end of the capillaries the blood pressure is
high enough $\left\{ \begin{array}{l} \textit{to force } \text{water} \\ \textit{for water to be } \text{forced} \end{array} \right\}$ into the tissue fluid.

Now change sentences (c), (e), (f) and (h) into the second form.

Section 3   Reading

10. Read the passage and choose a title for it:

If you think a title is not suitable, say whether it is too general, too limited, or not sufficiently accurate.

a) Lack and excess of oxygen c) Oxygen deficiencies
b) The effects of no oxygen   d) Obstructions of the respiratory system

The term anoxia literally means without oxygen and is commonly used to indicate conditions in which there is a shortage of oxygen. It is more appropriate to refer to a condition of too little oxygen as hypoxia. There are four commonly defined causes for lack of sufficient oxygen for the cells of the body, which will be
5 stated in the commonly used terms.
Anoxic anoxia, or hypoxic hypoxia, refers to decreased oxygen saturation of blood haemoglobin because of insufficient oxygen in the alveolar air. It is associated with low tension of oxygen in the arterial blood. This condition will be produced by obstructions of lung passages or situations where the
10 oxygen supply is inadequate.
The second type of anoxia is anaemic anoxia which occurs in individuals whose haemoglobin content is too low to carry the required amount of oxygen. The oxygen tension will be normal but there will be a shortage of oxygen carried by the blood due to the lack of haemoglobin.
15 The third type of anoxia is stagnant anoxia. This is due to the blood flowing too slowly round the circulation. Although the oxygen tension and oxygen content leaving the lungs are normal, the supplies of fresh oxygen are delivered too slowly to provide the tissues with sufficient oxygen.
The fourth type of anoxia is histotoxic anoxia, of which cyanide poisoning is
20 the only important example. The cyanide destroys the enzyme system of the cells and prevents their utilisation of the oxygen present in the blood.
Anoxia is more dangerous than asphyxia, in which not enough oxygen reaches the tissues and carbon dioxide is not expelled quickly enough. The accumulation of carbon dioxide produces a marked stimulation in respiration. In pure anoxia,
25 however, although respiratory stimulation may initially be produced, there is no accumulation of carbon dioxide and in severe cases respiration subsequently ceases altogether.

The following sentences have been omitted from the passage. Say which sentence each should follow:

e) This type of anoxia can also be caused by carbon monoxide poisoning, because this gas forms a bond with haemoglobin (carboxyhaemoglobin) leaving less haemoglobin available to transport oxygen.

73

f) This will occur in cases where there is reduced cardiac output or arterial obstruction locally.

g) These include insufficient partial pressure of oxygen, such as occurs at high altitudes, and breathing a gas mixture which contains insufficient oxygen.

h) This is a condition which can arise when, for example, one is breathing in a confined space so that the expired air is re-inhaled.

11. Copy this table and indicate whether or not the four situations described below are valid for each type of anoxia by putting a tick or a cross:

	Anoxic	Anaemic	Stagnant	Histotoxic
sufficient O_2 in lungs				
sufficient O_2 content of blood				
sufficient O_2 reaches tissues				
sufficient O_2 metabolised				

These diagrams show the causes of the different types of anoxia. Match the letters A to J with the phrases (a) to (j) below:

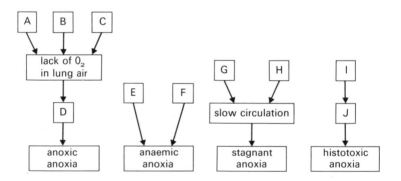

a) insufficient blood haemoglobin
b) inability of cell enzymes to metabolise O_2
c) respiratory blockage
d) CO bonding with haemoglobin
e) insufficient haemoglobin O_2 content
f) cyanide poisoning
g) living on a mountain
h) decreased cardiac output
i) inhaling air deficient in O_2
j) arterial blockage

Section 4 Listening

12. Copy the table below. Listen to the passage and complete the table using the following phrases:

an inadequate intake of folic acid
niacin deprivation
a lack of vitamin C
haemorrhage, bleeding gums
toxic effects

a prolonged shortage of vitamin C
a prolonged deficiency of thiamin
megaloblastic anaemia
skin changes, diarrhoea
beri-beri

DEFICIENCY	EFFECT	DISEASE
A shortage of vitamin A	changes in epithelium	xerophthalmia (eye dryness)
An excessive intake of vitamin A		
	disorder of carbohydrate metabolism	
		pellagra
	disturbance of DNA synthesis and red cell formation	
	defective formation of collagen fibres of connective tissue slow wound healing abnormal bone formation	
		scurvy

Now look at this example and then complete the sentences below:

In cases of xerophthalmia there is $\left\{\begin{array}{l}too\ little \\ not\ enough\end{array}\right\}$ vitamin A

for $\left\{\begin{array}{l}normal \\ healthy \\ proper\end{array}\right\}$ $\left\{\begin{array}{l}development \\ formation\end{array}\right\}$ of epithelium.

a) In cases of beri-beri ....
b) A dietary deficiency of folic acid may cause megaloblastic anaemia in which
....
c) In cases of pellagra ....
d) In cases of scurvy ....

Unit 8 Process 3 Cause and Effect

Section 1 Presentation

1. Read this:

(**Note:** the information is from the previous unit.)

$$A \left\{ \begin{array}{l} causes \\ produces \\ results\ in \\ leads\ to \end{array} \right\} B$$

Example: Lack of vitamin C *causes* defective collagen fibre formation.
Respiratory blockage *results in* alveolar oxygen deficiency.

Match these:

a) An excessive intake of vit. A produces	malformation of erythrocytes.
b) Folic acid deficiency causes	scurvy.
c) Thiamin deficiency results in	symptoms of toxicity.
d) Shortage of niacin produces	blindness.
e) Prolonged vit. C deficiency leads to	inflammation of the skin.
f) Vitamin A deficiency can lead to	disorders of carbohydrate metabolism.

$$B \left\{ \begin{array}{l} is\ caused\ by \\ is\ produced\ by \\ results\ from \\ occurs\ as\ a\ result\ of \end{array} \right\} A$$

Example: Defective collagen fibre formation *is caused by* vit. C deficiency.
Lack of alveolar oxygen may *result from* respiratory blockage.

Match these:

g) Histotoxic anoxia results from	carbon monoxide poisoning.
h) Respiratory stimulation in asphyxia occurs as a result of	a deficiency of oxygen in the lungs.
i) Lack of oxygen in the blood when the haemoglobin level is normal is produced by	carbon dioxide accumulation.
j) A lack of oxygen in the lungs may result from	a lack of haemoglobin in the blood.
k) Anaemic anoxia can be caused by	the destruction of the oxygen metabolising enzymes in the cells.
l) Anaemic anoxia may be produced by	insufficient partial pressure of oxygen in the air inhaled.

2. Read this:

When there is more than one possible cause, we use 'may' or 'can'.

Examples: Anoxia *may* be caused by a deficiency in the oxygen supply.
Anoxia *can* occur as a result of lack of available haemoglobin.
Anoxia *may* be produced by other factors.

If, however, the cause is certain, the present simple is usually used.

Example: Histotoxic anoxia is caused by the destruction of the cell enzyme system.

Now complete these sentences:

a) Pellagra ...... niacin deprivation.
b) Stagnant anoxia ...... slow blood circulation.
c) Slow blood circulation ...... a localised obstruction of the arteries.
d) Changes in the epithelial tissue of the skin ...... vit. A deficiency.

3. Look and read:

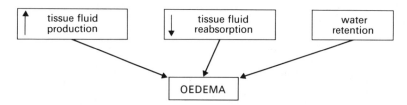

Oedema can be *caused by* increased production of tissue fluid.
Oedema may be *due to* decreased reabsorption of tissue fluid.
Oedema may occur *because of* water retention in the tissue fluid.

Compare the following diagrams with that in Unit 7, exercise 9 and add labels:

increased capillary pressure   reduced osmotic pressure   sodium retention

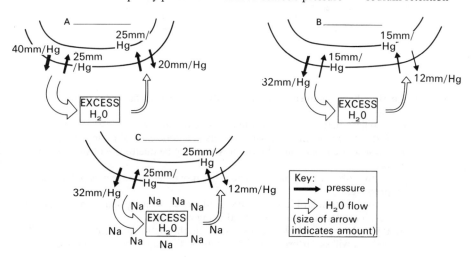

Now complete these:

  a) Increased tissue fluid production may be due to ......
  b) Less tissue fluid may be reabsorbed because of ......
  c) Water retention in the tissues ......

Match four of the following diagrams with D to G below:

d) increased arteriolar b.p.

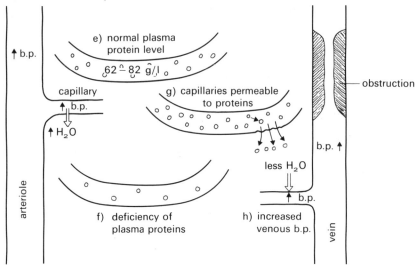

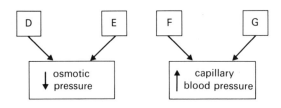

Now say whether these statements are true or false. Correct the false statements.

  i) Capillary permeability to proteins is due to a decrease in osmotic pressure.
  j) A decrease in osmotic pressure results in a deficiency of plasma proteins.
  k) An increase in capillary blood pressure may be due to the obstruction of a vein.
  l) Venous obstruction may also occur because of an increase in capillary blood pressure.
  m) A rise in arteriolar blood pressure produces a rise in capillary blood pressure which results in excess tissue fluid being produced.
  n) If plasma proteins leak into the tissue fluid through a damaged capillary wall, oedema will occur because of the reduction in capillary blood pressure.

4. Read this:

$$\left\{ \begin{array}{ll} \text{A } causes & \text{B} \\ \text{B } is\ caused\ by & \text{A} \\ \text{B } is\ due\ to & \text{A} \end{array} \right\}$$ A is the CAUSE
                                    B is the EFFECT

Answer these questions:

       a) What is one cause of oedema?
       b) What is an effect of haemoglobin deficiency?
       c) What is the cause of pellagra?
       d) What is one effect of venous obstruction?
       e) What is the cause of beri-beri?
       f) What is a result of an inadequate intake of vitamin A?

Complete these:

       g) The wounds of a vitamin C deficient patient will heal slowly because of ....
       h) Oedema occurs in cases of capillary damage due to ....
       i) Asphyxia is less dangerous than anoxia because of the ...... due to ....

Write two full sentences about each of the following, using it once as a cause and
once as an effect:

       j) a reduction in osmotic pressure
       k) an increase in capillary blood pressure
       l) lack of oxygen in the lungs
       m) inability of cell enzymes to metabolise oxygen

Now write CAUSE or EFFECT above the appropriate phrases in each sentence you
have written:

Copy and complete this diagram:

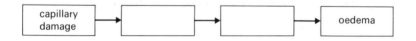

5. Look at this:

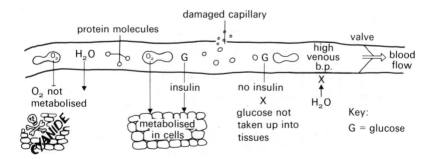

79

Capillary walls $\begin{cases} \textit{allow} \text{ water molecules } \textit{to pass} \text{ through.} \\ \textit{let} \text{ water molecules } \textit{pass} \text{ through.} \end{cases}$

Capillary walls *prevent* $\begin{cases} \text{protein molecules (from) pass}\textit{ing}\text{ through.} \\ \text{the passage of protein molecules.} \end{cases}$

High venous b.p. *prevents* water *being drawn* back into the blood.

Complete these sentences:

    a) Damaged capillaries allow ....
    b) Insulin allows ....
    c) Valves in venous blood vessels let ....
    d) Valves prevent ....
    e) Lack of insulin prevents ....
    f) The presence of cyanide in the tissues prevents ....
    g) A semipermeable membrane allows ...... but prevents ....

Section 2   Development

6. Read and look:

The activities of the organs of the body are controlled in two ways, by hormones and nerves. Hormones are chemical substances, produced by endocrine glands, which circulate in the blood and bring about effects in distant organs.

     The posterior pituitary gland, for example, produces two hormones, one of
5 which, antidiuretic hormone (ADH), regulates the reabsorption of water by the kidney tubules. If the body is short of water, more ADH will be released into the blood. Since ADH controls water reabsorption in the kidneys, an increase in ADH will produce an increase in the amount of water reabsorbed so that less urine will be produced.

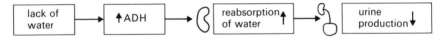

Now look at this diagram and complete the following passage:

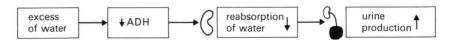

If, on the other hand, there is ...... water in the body, ... will be released into the blood. Consequently the water reabsorption rate ......, thereby increasing
....

7. Look at this:

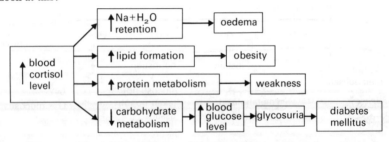

Match sentences a) to d) with A to D below:

    a) The adrenal hormone, cortisol, has an effect opposite to that of insulin
       (which promotes the metabolism of glucose).
    b) Proteins have to be broken down to amino acids to form this glucose.
    c) Another feature of this syndrome is increased lipid formation and storage.
    d) In addition, excess cortisol causes retention of sodium and therefore water.

    A. Consequently there is loss of muscle, leading to weakness and tiredness.
    B. As a result patients often have the 'moon face' produced by oedema.
    C. Therefore an excess of cortisol causes an increase in the formation and
       storage of glucose (gluconeogenesis).
    D. Hence we see the characteristic 'buffalo hump' (accumulation of fat at the
       lower part of the bottom of the neck).

Now match e) to i) with E to I. Then rearrange the combined sentences to form a paragraph.

    e) This excess of cortisol will have the effect of increasing the formation and
       storage of carbohydrate and reducing its metabolism in the cells ....
    f) If the level exceeds 180 mg glucose per 100 ml blood ....
    g) If the secretion of cortisol from the adrenal gland increases ....
    h) This form of diabetes, however, cannot be treated with insulin ....
    i) This alteration in carbohydrate metabolism means that glucose is being
       added to the blood but not being used up.

    E. Consequently the blood glucose level rises.
    F. the blood cortisol level will rise.
    G. since cortisol inhibits the action of insulin.
    H. because it is due to an excess of cortisol and is therefore insulin-resistant.
    I. glucose will appear in the urine, thereby indicating diabetes mellitus.

8. Look at these different ways of expressing cause and effect:

Since
Because } carbohydrate is not metabolised, the blood glucose level rises.
As

Carbohydrate is not metabolised. *Therefore* / *Consequently* / *Hence* / *As a result* } the blood glucose level rises.

Carbohydrate is not metabolised { *with the result that* blood glucose rises. / *thereby* / *thus* } *raising* the blood glucose level.

{ *If* the secretion of cortisol increases, the blood cortisol level will rise. / The secretion of cortisol may increase, *in which case* the blood cortisol level will rise.

Now change the sentences you have formed in exercise 7 to alternative forms using the connecting words given:

    Example: a) as → As cortisol has an effect opposite to that of insulin, an excess
                 of cortisol causes an increase in the formation and storage of
                 glucose.

b) since	d) thus	f) because	h) consequently
c) as	e) therefore	g) in which case	

Section 3 Reading

9. Read the passage and choose a suitable title:

(say why the others are not suitable)

Diabetes
Diabetes Mellitus

The causes of diabetes
The effects of diabetes

Diabetes mellitus is a clinical syndrome involving a variety of metabolic disorders characterised by hyperglycaemia. The hyperglycaemia results from the fact that insulin secreted by the pancreas is either insufficient in amount or ineffective in action and arises from two main sources, namely a reduced rate of
5 removal of glucose from the blood by the peripheral tissues and an increased rate of release of glucose from the liver into the circulation.

As a result of the hyperglycaemia large amounts of glucose are excreted in the urine. Because of the increase of glucose in the kidney filtrate water reabsorption is prevented. In this way the volume of urine is markedly increased in diabetes;
10 this in turn leads to loss of water and minerals, thereby making the diabetic very thirsty so that he drinks large amounts of fluid (without however satisfying his thirst).

Answer these:

a) What is the cause of diabetes mellitus?
b) What is the primary clinical sign of diabetes mellitus?
c) What is hyperglycaemia due to?
d) Why does glycosuria occur?
e) What are the effects of glycosuria?

Complete this diagram using the following terms:

f) glycosuria
g) hepatic overproduction of glucose
h) hyperglycaemia
i) peripheral underutilisation of glucose
j) polydipsia
k) polyuria

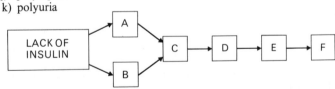

10. Read this:

In other patients, however, further features develop if treatment is not begun quickly enough. The tissues, although receiving liberal supplies of glucose from the blood, are unable to utilise it effectively in the absence of insulin and so the diabetic feels weak and tired. This causes two main compensatory mechanisms to
5 operate, both of which lead to loss of body tissue. Protein is broken down to provide energy and fat replaces carbohydrate as a fuel. Since the fat must be transferred from the body stores to the liver to be broken down, the fat content of both the blood and the liver is increased; thus a plasma sample from an untreated diabetic is often fatty.

10　In severe cases of diabetes the disproportionate metabolism of fat results in the overproduction of ketone bodies* (acetone, acetoacetic acid, and β-hydroxy-butyric acid) leading to ketonaemia and ketonuria. Furthermore, as acetoacetic and β-hydroxybutyric acids are produced faster than they can be metabolised, the patient develops acidaemia, one of the effects of which is to stimulate breath-

15　ing so that clinically 'air hunger' is observed.

* Ketone bodies are intermediate products in the breakdown of fats to CO_2 and H_2O: a process only completed if carbohydrates are being metabolised.

Look at this:

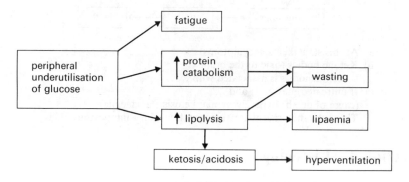

Explain each of the terms in the diagram (with reference to the passage).

Answer these:

a) What are the 'further features' referred to in line 1?
b) Why can the muscles of a diabetic not provide enough energy?
c) What is the cause of loss of body tissue in a diabetic?
d) Why is there an increase in protein catabolism?
e) What will the effect of this be on wound healing if that process requires proteins?
f) Why does the increase in lipolysis affect the blood?
g) What does 'disproportionate metabolism of fat' refer to?
h) How does an increase in lipolysis lead to ketosis?
i) Why does an excess of ketone bodies produce excess *acid* in the blood?
j) Why is hyperventilation sometimes observed in a diabetic?

11. Select and arrange four of these phrases as paragraph headings for the two passages:

a) Effects of hyperglycaemia
b) Treatment of the further features
c) Incidence of ketosis
d) Consequences of poor glucose utilisation
e) What is 'diabetes mellitus'?
f) Effects of increased lipolysis
g) Hyperglycaemia

12. Using the diagram and the notes below, write the next paragraph:

(**Note**: don't forget the glossary at the back of the book.)

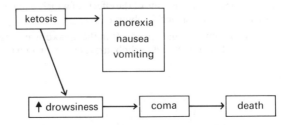

a) At this stage/ketosis/(symptoms)
b) Ketone bodies toxic to the brain
   ∴ keto-acidosis is associated with ......
c) If untreated/may ...... and ......
   (cause of death: hyperglycaemia, ketosis + acidaemia)
d) This outcome/prevent/treatment with insulin + intravenous fluids

Section 4   Listening

13. As you listen to the passage, make a brief note of:

    a) the three methods of treatment
    b) the effect of sulphonylureas
    c) the effect of diguanides

Listen again and answer these questions:

    d) What is the effect of a controlled diet?
    e) Why do some diabetics require injections of insulin?
    f) What is the result of injecting insulin?
    g) What is the effect of hypoglycaemic drugs?
    h) What does 'obese' mean?
    i) Using information from the reading passages as well as the listening passage, complete this diagrammatic summary of the action of hypoglycaemic drugs:

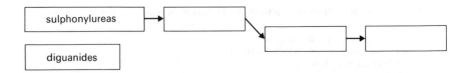

Unit 9   Measurement 3 Proportion

Section 1   Presentation

1. Look at this:

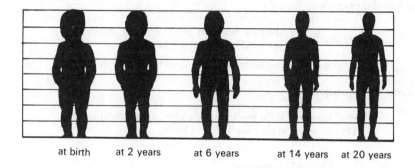

| at birth | at 2 years | at 6 years | at 14 years | at 20 years |

Changes in the proportions of the human body during growth

From the diagram we can observe that the head size at birth is nearly 25 % of the total body size.

Answer these questions:

a) When is the head size about 18 % of the total?
b) When is it approximately 12 % of the total?
c) At what point is leg length about 25 % of the total body length?
d) When is it nearly 50 %?

Look at this example:

At birth { the *ratio* {of / between} head size {to / and} total body size is about 1 : 4 (one to four).
the head to body size *ratio* is approximately 1 : 4 (and at its highest).

Answer these questions:

e) When is the head to body size ratio about 1 : 8 (at its lowest)?
f) When is the leg to body length ratio at its highest, and when is it at its lowest?
g) What are the approximate ratios at these times?
h) What is the approximate ratio of body length to arm length at 6 years? (Careful!)

From the previous statements we can deduce that the head is
{ *relatively* / *proportionately* } bigger at birth than at the age of 20.

(**Note:** The head is of course larger at 20; but as a proportion of percentage of the total body size at that time it is smaller.)

85

Answer these questions:

     i) When are the legs longest in proportion to the whole body?
     j) When are the arms proportionately longest?
     k) When is the neck relatively thickest?
     l) When is it proportionately thinnest?
     m) Is the waist proportionately bigger or smaller at birth than at 20?
     n) What can you observe about the length and thickness of the legs in early
          childhood and at 20 years?

Look at this example:

During childhood $\begin{cases}\text{the head becomes } \textit{proportionately} \text{ small} er. \\ \text{the head to body size } \textit{ratio decreases.}\end{cases}$

i.e. the size of the head decreases relative to the size of the body.

Answer these questions:

     o) What happens to the legs between early and late childhood?
     p) What happens to the neck between birth and 20 years?

Section 2   Development

**2. Look at this diagram which shows how the rate of growth is affected by hormones in the
body:**

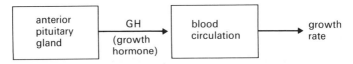

Rate of growth $\quad$ $\begin{cases}\textit{is controlled by} \\ \textit{is determined by} \\ \textit{depends on}\end{cases}$ the presence of GH in the blood.
The blood GH level $\qquad$ the rate of GH secretion from the
$\qquad\qquad\qquad\qquad\qquad\qquad$ anterior pituitary.

Look at this:

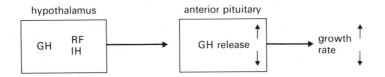

Growth hormone releasing factor *promotes* growth hormone release.
Growth hormone inhibiting hormone *inhibits* growth hormone release.

Complete these:

     a) The release of GH ...... secretions of the hypothalamus.
     b) By secreting GH-Releasing Factor the hypothalamus promotes the release
         of ....
     c) By ...... GH-Inhibiting Hormone, ... (inhibit) ....

Read this:

> The release of GH is *directly proportional* to secretion of GH–RF.
>   The more GH–RF is secreted, the more GH is released, (and, conversely, the less GH–RF is secreted, the less GH is released).

– If GH–RF is secreted, more GH will be released by the anterior pituitary.

> The release of GH is *inversely proportional* to secretion of GH–IH.
> – The more GH–IH is secreted, the less GH will be released.

– If GH–IH is secreted, less GH will be released, (and, conversely, if GH–IH is not secreted, more GH will be released).

Say whether these statements are true or false. Correct the false statements.

   d) The release of GH depends on growth rate.
   e) The hypothalamus determines the level of GH in the blood.
   f) Growth rate is inversely proportional to the level of GH in the blood.
   g) The more GH–RF is secreted by the hypothalamus, the faster is the growth rate.
   h) If the secretion of GH into the blood decreases, it will be due to the release of GH–RF from the hypothalamus.
   i) The hypothalamus determines the release of the anterior pituitary gland.
   j) If the hypothalamus releases more GH–IH, the growth rate will increase.
   k) The hypothalamus inhibits growth rate by increasing the secretion of GH–IH.
   l) By releasing GH, the anterior pituitary gland inhibits the growth rate.
   m) GH release from the anterior pituitary is inversely proportional to the amount of GH–IH received from the hypothalamus.

3. Look at this:

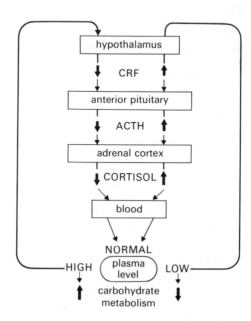

Key:
CRF = Corticotrophin
        Releasing
        Factor

ACTH = Adreno
          cortico –
          trophic –
          Hormone

Complete these sentences, or construct sentences from the notes given:

    a) The release of cortisol from the adrenal cortex depends on ....
    b) The rate of carbohydrate metabolism is determined by ....
    c) The secretion of CRF promotes ....
    d) The release of ACTH is inhibited by ....
    e) (ACTH/rate of carbohydrate metabolism)
    f) If more CRF is secreted by the hypothalamus ....
    g) If the rate of carbohydrate metabolism decreases ....
    h) Cortisol release is directly proportional to ....
    i) The more cortisol is released from the adrenal cortex ...... and, conversely, ...
    j) The release of CRF ...... to the plasma cortisol level.

Read this:

If the cortisol level rises, the hypothalamus acts to restore it to normal by stimulating the release of ACTH.

Write similar sentences using these notes:

    k) growth rate ↑/hypothalamus/GH–IH
    l) too much carbohydrate – metabolise/hypothalamus/ACTH

4. Say whether the relationship between the following pairs is one of direct or inverse proportion and write a sentence expressing that relationship:

(Do not use the same pattern more than twice.)

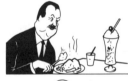

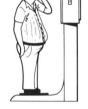

a) food intake/body weight

b) exercise/body weight

c) blood insulin level/ utilisation of glucose in tissues

d) insulin level/blood glucose level

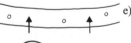

e) plasma protein level/ osmotic pressure

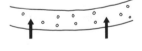

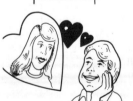

f) emotional excitement/ heart rate

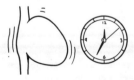

Section 3   Reading

5. Read this passage and answer this question:

What is hyperpnoea?

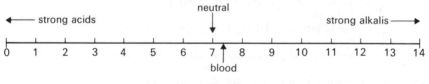

Blood pH scale

The pH scale is a measure of the concentration of hydrogen ions in the blood, or in other words the relative acidity or alkalinity of the blood. Life is possible only if the blood is kept within a range of alkalinity corresponding to a pH of between 7·35 and 7·45. For the pH to be kept constant at this level, the relative con-
5 centrations of the main base component, bicarbonate, and the main acid component, carbonic acid, must be maintained in the ratio 20:1.

Acidosis arises as a result of an increase in the proportion of acids in the blood, whether due to a body depletion of the base bicarbonate or to an increase in acid production or ingestion. Sulphuric acid, for example, may be ingested in
10 cheap lemonade, or an abnormal amount of acetoacetic acid may be produced in a diabetic. In such cases, the excess acid is neutralised, or buffered, by bi-carbonates in the blood. This means that the ratio of bicarbonate to carbonic acid becomes less than 20:1 (in other words the blood becomes more acid, or the pH falls). This tends to stimulate respiration. Since the concentration of car-
15 bonic acid in the plasma is determined by the partial pressure of carbon dioxide (P_{CO_2}) in the alveoli, the hyperpnoea tends to reduce the level of carbonic acid in the blood by reducing the P_{CO_2} in the lungs. The effect of this is to restore the bicarbonate to acid ratio to its normal level of 20:1.

Answer these questions:

    a) Is the blood normally acid, alkaline or neutral?
    b) Is there more carbonic acid or bicarbonate in the blood?
    c) The more bicarbonate there is in the blood, the lower the pH falls. Is this true?
    d) If the normal value for plasma bicarbonate is 22–24 mmol/l, what will the normal value be for carbonic acid?
    e) What does the plasma carbonic acid level depend on?
    f) What will be the effects of vigorous exercise (in which large amounts of lactic acid are produced)?
    g) What will happen to blood pH in severe cases of diarrhoea, considering that one of the substances excreted in the faeces is sodium bicarbonate?
    h) How does hyperpnoea affect blood pH?
    i) Severe and continued vomiting is associated with loss of hydrochloric acid and can result in carbohydrate deficiency and a consequent increase in lipolysis, producing abnormal amounts of acetoacetic acid. Will acidosis result?
    j) What do you think the subject of the next paragraph would be?

6. Rearrange these notes to form a summary of the passage:

a) Excess acid buffered by bicarbonate
b) → reduction in lung PCO_2
c) e.g. H_2SO_4 in lemonade, keto-acids in diabetes
d) → bicarbonate – acid ratio normal
e) Acidosis = ↑ proportion of acid in blood
f) → ↓ H_2CO_3
g) ∴ less bicarbonate; $HCO_3 : H_2CO_3$ ↓ ($<20:1$)
h) → hyperpnoea
i) caused by ↑ acid production/ingestion, or ↓ plasma base

> KEY
> → results in
> ∴ therefore

Now, using these notes, write a paragraph about alkalosis:

Alkalosis = relatively more bases
e.g. abnormal loss of HCl in prolonged/severe vomiting
    ingestion of large amounts of $Na(HCO_3)_2$

Plasma HCO_3 ↑
∴ $HCO_3 : H_2CO_3$ ↑ ($>20:1$)   i.e. ......
    → respiration ↓   (use the verb *depress*.)
        → blood CO_2 ↑ (∴ H_2CO_3 ↑)
            → $20:1$ (but with respiration ↓)

Section 4   Listening

7. Copy this diagram and try to complete it as you listen to the passage:

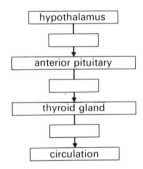

Hormone control of metabolic rate

As you listen to the passage a second time, try to complete these notes on 'mechanism of thyroid function and its control':

Thyroid gland: function –
    This depends on ......
    TSH secretion controlled by ......
    TRH ↑ →
Blood thyroxine level ...... proportional to ......
    – ...... by 'negative feedback mechanism'
        i.e. blood thyroxine ↓ →
            (or ...... proportional to ......)

Using your completed notes, write a paragraph about the subject.

Unit C Revision

1. Read this and complete the sentences where necessary:

Concentration of a solution refers to the amount of a substance (or substances) in a fluid. In medicine it is usually referred to as *osmolarity* and expressed in millimoles per litre (mmol/l).

$$\text{millimoles per litre} = \frac{\text{milligrams per litre}}{\text{molecular weight}}$$

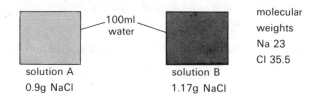

solution A	100ml water	solution B	molecular weights
0.9g NaCl		1.17g NaCl	Na 23
			Cl 35.5

The osmolarity of solution A is $\frac{\text{(mg.NaCl/1.H}_2\text{O)}}{\text{(mol.wt.NaCl)}}$ $\frac{9000}{58\cdot5} = \frac{154 \text{ mmol/1}}{\text{(approx.)}}$

a) The osmolarity of solution B is ....
b) Therefore the concentration of solution B is (higher/lower) than that of A.
c) i.e. The more molecules of a substance in a solution, ...
   Furthermore, each molecule exerts osmotic pressure (in other words, osmotic pressure depends on the number of molecules).
d) Consequently osmotic pressure is ...... to osmolarity.
e) In other words, the lower the osmolarity, ...
f) Or, the more molecules in a solution, ... (osmotic pressure).

2. Look at this:

Filtration, reabsorption and excretion of ions and water by an adult man with a glomerular filtration rate of 180 1/24 hr.

	Plasma concentration	Amount filtered	Amount excreted	Amount reabsorbed	Per cent reabsorbed
	(mmol/l)	(mmol/24 h)	(mmol/24 h)	(mmol/24 h)	
Sodium	142	25,560	250	25,310	99·0
Chloride	100	18,000	250	17,750	98·6
Bicarbonate	28	5,040	2	5,038	>99·9
Potassium	4	720	120	600	83·3
	(kg/1)	(kg/24 h)	(kg/24 h)	(kg/24 h)	
Water	0·93	167·4	1·5	165·9	99·1

Answer these questions:

a) How much sodium is reabsorbed per day?
b) What proportion of sodium is reabsorbed per day?
c) Which ion is present in the blood in the highest proportion?
d) What is the plasma osmolarity of bicarbonate?
e) What is the ratio of potassium to bicarbonate in the plasma?
f) What is the ratio of filtered chloride to chloride excreted?
g) What is the ratio of reabsorbed to filtered potassium?
h) What is the ratio between the amount of chloride filtered and the amount of sodium?

Say whether these are true or false. Correct the false ones.

i) There is proportionately more sodium excreted every 24 hours than chloride.
j) The kidneys reabsorb relatively more water than sodium.
k) Proportionately more sodium is reabsorbed than bicarbonate.
l) The ratio of excreted to reabsorbed chloride is lower than the ratio between excreted and reabsorbed potassium.

3. Read this passage and choose a title for it. Say why the other titles are not suitable:

Pituitary function   Effects of ADH secretion
ADH   ADH control
ADH function   ADH secretion

The posterior pituitary gland also produces the antidiuretic hormone (ADH). Like oxytocin it is a peptide, but it has a molecular weight of 1102. Its principal function is the control of water reabsorption in the distal convoluted tubule and the collecting ducts of the kidney.
5   In large doses ADH causes contraction of smooth muscle, particularly in the blood vessels of the skin and in the splanchnic bed; this leads to a rise in blood pressure.
Secretion of ADH provides a homeostatic mechanism to maintain the osmolarity of body fluids within a relatively narrow range. Two main types of re-
10 ceptor have been postulated: hypothalamic receptors sensitive to changes in osmolarity (osmoreceptors) and baroreceptors, sensitive to changes in blood volume, which are situated in the large thoracic blood vessels. The latter are linked to the hypothalamus by the vagus nerve. ADH is secreted continuously, basal plasma levels being 1 to 5 ng/l. When there is an increase in plasma
15 osmolarity due to dehydration, or a fall in blood volume due to haemorrhage, the secretion of ADH increases and the resulting water retention restores the osmolarity or blood volume to normal.
On the other hand, a deficiency of ADH (which is a more common condition) leads to diabetes insipidus. Large volumes of urine are passed each day and the
20 patient is excessively thirsty. The urine is very dilute. Before the days of chemical tests, the standard method of testing urine was to taste it. In diabetes insipidus the urine was tasteless or insipid; in diabetes mellitus, where there is also an increase in urine production, the urine was sweet to the taste.

4. Insert these sentences/clauses in suitable places in the passage:

a) Conversely a decrease in plasma osmolarity, or a rise in blood volume, will lead to a decrease in ADH secretion and the resulting diuresis will restore normal levels.
b) since it contained glucose.

c) It does this by increasing the permeability of the luminal membrane.
d) There is a clinically recognisable syndrome, involving a fall in plasma sodium, which may be observed if secretion is excessive.
e) The effects of ADH on smooth muscle are probably not important in physiological concentrations.
f) hence the name of this condition.

5. Put the following in the order in which they occur in the passage:

a) Normal levels of ADH.
b) Effects of ADH lack.
c) Structure of ADH.
d) Balance of ADH secretion and normal concentrations.
e) Control of ADH secretion.
f) Function of ADH.
g) Effects of excess ADH secretion.

6. Copy this diagram and complete it by inserting the symbols ↑ and ↓ in the appropriate places:

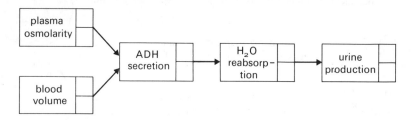

7. Complete these sentences, or write a sentence to express the relationship or idea indicated in the notes given:

a) Secretion of ADH depends on ....
b) The more ADH is secreted ....
c) Plasma osmolarity is ...... to dehydration.
d) (blood volume/ADH secretion)
e) (ADH secretion/water reabsorption)   (2 sentences)
f) (ADH secretion/urine production)
g) (an effect of haemorrhage)
h) (a cause of diuresis)
i) In diabetes insipidus there is not enough ADH for ....
j) Dehydration causes ...... (osmolarity) by ....
k) ADH controls ...... by ....
l) ADH acts on ...... to ....

Unit 10 Measurement 4 Frequency and Probability

Section 1 Presentation

1. Look at the sentences expressing the frequency of occurrence of various signs and symptoms of influenza. Complete the subsequent sentences in the same way:

In cases of influenza, a dry cough $\left\{\begin{array}{l}almost\ always\\ almost\ invariably\end{array}\right\}$ occurs.
A dry cough is present in *nearly all* cases of 'flu.

...... backache (or an ache in some other part of the body) is *usually* observed.
Backache or some other body ache ...... *most* cases of 'flu.

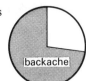

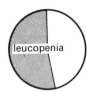

...... leucopenia *frequently* occurs.
Leucopenia ...... *many* cases of 'flu.

...... is *sometimes* observed.
...... in *some* cases ....

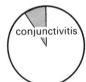

...... *occasionally* ....
...... *a few* cases ....

...... *seldom/rarely* ....
...... *very few* ....

...... *never* ....
...... *no* ....

Now make similar sentences about the signs and symptoms of the following two diseases:

PNEUMONIA

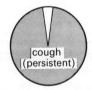

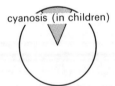

cyanosis (in children)

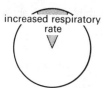

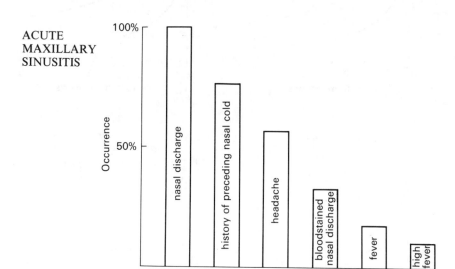

2. **Look at these ways of predicting what will happen:**

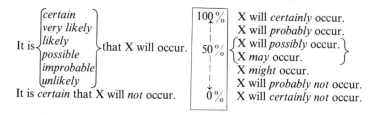

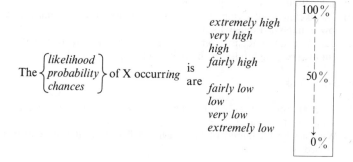

Now look at these graphs, which show the annual survival rates for different forms of cancer (in England):

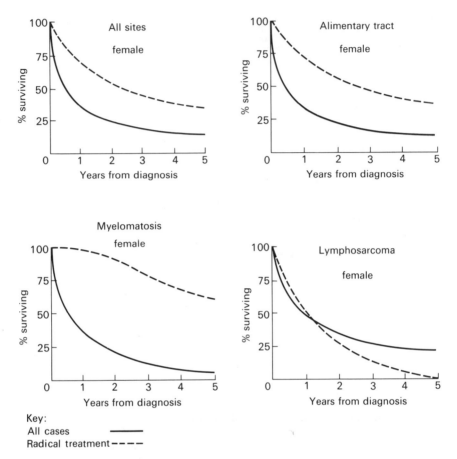

Key:
All cases ————
Radical treatment ————

Choose the correct word/phrase to complete these sentences:

a) A female patient with cancer will (certainly/possibly/probably not) survive for five years without radical treatment.
b) If a woman has a cancer completely removed, it is (likely/possible/unlikely) that she will live five years.
c) If a woman has a cancer in the alimentary tract, it is (very likely/likely/unlikely) that she will die within five years.
d) The likelihood of a woman surviving five years with myelomatosis is (fairly low/unlikely/extremely low).
e) But the chances for myelomatosis cases where radical treatment is carried out are (very high/fairly high/fairly low).

Answer these questions:

f) What are the chances of surviving for five years for a woman with cancer of the alimentary tract?
g) What is the likelihood of her surviving five years if radical treatment is carried out?

h) What is the probability of surviving for two years after radical treatment of myelomatosis?

i) Is it likely that a patient will survive five years if she has lymphosarcoma?

j) How likely is a patient to live for four years after radical treatment of lymphosarcoma?

Complete these:

k) If a woman has ......, there is a 1 in 2 chance of her surviving five years. (a 1 in 2 chance = a 50% chance)

l) The chances of ...... five years in cases of lymphosarcoma are about ......, unless radical treatment ......, in which case ...... are zero.

m) The chances of ...... are only about 1 in 15, unless ......, in which case ....

Read this:

The *prognosis* for myelomatosis is very bad. However, for cases involving radical treatment the prognosis is fairly good.

The prognosis for cancer cases treated radically *tends to* be better (i.e. is usually better), though there are exceptions, such as lymphosarcoma.

Make similar statements about other diseases.

Section 2   Development

3. Read this short passage about the clinical features of renal calculi (kidney stones):

There is a characteristic pain over the kidney or ureter which nearly always becomes severe. It is usually fairly constant (severe intermittent pain is, in fact, rare). The pain is occasionally aggravated by deep breathing or movement. In a few cases, stones are passed in the urine. Haematuria is almost invariably
5 present and can often be seen by the patient. Frequency may occur and the patient sometimes has difficulty urinating. Vomiting is common.

Put the following symptoms in approximate order of frequency of occurrence.
Group together symptoms which occur with approximately equal frequency:

a) constant severe pain   e) macroscopic haematuria
b) intermittent severe pain   f) dysuria
c) passage of calculi   g) frequency
d) microscopic haematuria   h) vomiting

Write statements of prediction, using the words given, as in this example:

stones/pass/urine

The likelihood of stones being passed in the urine is low (very low).

i) pain/cause/urination
j) vomiting/observe
k) pain/intermittent
l) pain/aggravate/breathing or movement
m) blood/pass/urine
n) the blood which is passed/sufficient to ...... by the patient

4. Read this:

A *characteristic* feature of a disease is one which is usually or nearly always present (although not invariably). It is the main feature, which is special to that disease, or is the feature most commonly associated with that illness.

Example: Periodic high fever is a characteristic feature of malaria.
Malaria is characterised by periodic high fever.

Match symptom with disease from these lists and write similar sentences:

a) haematuria	pellagra
b) skin lesions	diabetes
c) glycosuria	schistosomiasis

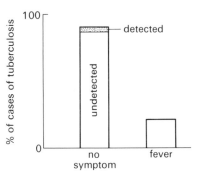

In tuberculosis, the characteristic feature is a lesion known as a tubercle. These lesions tend to heal by calcification (i.e. this is what generally happens, unless there are exceptional circumstances).

In the large majority of cases, the primary infection is symptomless, and passes unnoticed, unless there is a radiological examination (X-ray); but such close observation is seldom carried out.

Now with the help of the diagram, complete the paragraph below by selecting *one* suitable word/phrase from the list for each gap:

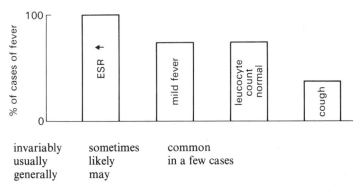

invariably	sometimes	common
usually	likely	in a few cases
generally	may	

...(d)... the primary infection produces a fever. It is ...(e)... mild, and lasts for no more than 7 to 14 days, but it ...(f)... be accompanied by other features of tuberculous infection. A slight dry cough is ...(g)... present; the leucocyte count is ...(h)... normal, but the erythrocyte sedimentation rate is ...(i)... raised.

Note how the use of 'not' with a negative adjective or adverb changes the meaning:

X is not impossible = X is possible
X is not uncommon = X is (fairly) common
X is not infrequent = X is (fairly) frequent

Say whether these statements concerning renal calculi are true or false:

j) It is not unusual for haematuria to be visible to the patient.
k) The passage of calculi is not uncommon.
l) Vomiting is not infrequently observed.

Section 3   Reading

5. Read this passage and choose the most suitable title for it:

Tuberculosis   The frequency of tuberculosis
Tuberculous lesions   The pathology of tuberculosis

The initial 'primary' tuberculous infection usually occurs in the lung but occasionally in the tonsil or in the alimentary tract, especially the ileo-caecal region. The primary infection differs from later infections in that the primary focus in lung, tonsil or bowel is almost invariably accompanied by a caseous
5   lesion in the regional lymph nodes, i.e. in the mediastinal, cervical or mesenteric groups respectively.

In most people the primary lesion and the associated lymph node lesion heal and calcify. In a few, healing (particularly of the lymph node lesion) is incomplete and surviving tubercle bacilli may under certain circumstances, such as a lower-
10 ing of the general health or an alteration of the balance between allergy and immunity, be discharged into the blood stream. Such patients may, in conse-quence, develop tuberculous lesions elsewhere in the body. The most common sites for 'haematogenous' lesions of this kind are the lungs, bones, joints and kidneys. Such lesions may develop months or even years after the primary
15 infection.

Rarely, a caseous tuberculous focus either at the site of the primary infection or, more commonly, in an associated lymph node ruptures into a vein and pro-duces acute dissemination of the disease throughout the body, a condition known as *acute miliary tuberculosis*. Tuberculous meningitis often accompanies
20 this condition.

Discuss to what extent these statements are true or not. Make them all as accurate as possible:

a) Primary foci are very common in the region of the bowels where the ileum joins the caecum.
b) All primary foci in the bowels have associated caseous lesions in the medi-astinal lymph nodes.
c) The discharge of tubercle bacilli into the blood stream is uncommon.
d) In cases where the general health is poor, tubercle bacilli are likely to be dis-charged into the blood.
e) Haematogenous lesions are very common.
f) The likelihood of a haematogenous lesion being found in the tonsil is high.
g) Acute miliary tuberculosis is a rare condition.
h) In cases of acute miliary tuberculosis, it is not uncommon for tuberculous meningitis to be found.

Complete these:

i) In the few cases where healing is incomplete, it is usually ...... which has not healed properly.
j) Most cases of acute miliary tuberculosis arise following the rupture of ....

6. Read the passage, copy and complete the diagram with the 6 appropriate labels from this list:

a) acquired immunity
b) diabetes mellitus
c) entry of tubercle bacillus into body
d) inadequate diet

e) low natural resistance
f) pregnancy
g) poor housing

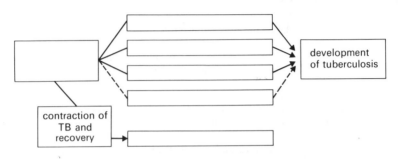

Aetiology of tuberculosis

The fact that tuberculosis is a specific infectious disease was first proved by Koch's discovery of the tubercle bacillus in 1882. However, entry of the bacillus into the body is not necessarily followed by a clinical illness, the development of which depends on several other factors.

5   The fact, for example, that certain races, such as Africans and Indians, and even certain regional groups, such as the inhabitants of the Western Isles of Scotland and of Ireland, are more likely to develop tuberculosis suggests that natural resistance varies from race to race and even from region to region. In contrast, although acquired immunity is not fully understood, it has been proved
10 that if a person contracts and recovers from a primary tuberculous infection he is less likely to develop active tuberculosis on subsequent exposure to the tubercle bacillus than a patient who has not previously been infected.

    Among other relevant factors, poor housing with its associated overcrowding has been shown to increase the risk of infection or reinfection with tuberculosis
15 and, while the exact part that diet plays is uncertain, it seems that a severe lack of protein and vitamins could be an important aetiological factor. In addition it is evident that conditions such as diabetes mellitus, gastrectomy and congenital heart disease, as well as treatment with corticosteroids, all make the development of tuberculosis more likely. Moreover it appears that pregnancy may have
20 an unfavourable effect on the course of untreated pulmonary tuberculosis.

7. Complete the following sentences:

a) While it is well known that tuberculosis is caused ......, it is also evident that this alone is not sufficient ......

b) Because of differences in ......, natural resistance to it is thought to ......

c) Although we do not yet completely understand ......, there is evidence that a person who ...... is ......

d) It has been demonstrated that poor housing ......, owing to its connection with ......

e) Although ...... understood, severe protein and vitamin deficiency is thought ......

f) The risk of developing tuberculosis is clearly ...... diabetes mellitus, while the course of the disease is probably ......

Section 4 Listening

8. Read these statements. Then listen to the passage about the treatment of tuberculosis and modify each statement to show how true it is using such phrases as:

it has been shown that	there is no evidence that ......
...... has proved that	it is thought that ......
there is evidence	it seems/appears ......
it is doubtful whether	...... probably ......
etc.	it would be a mistake to suppose that ......

a) Sanatorium treatment is unnecessary for tuberculosis.
b) No more tuberculosis cases occur in the families of home-treated patients than of those treated in a sanatorium.
c) The chemotherapy of tuberculosis is a straightforward matter.
d) Bronchoscopy is useful in the treatment of primary tuberculosis.
e) Bronchoscopy is useful in cases of obstructive emphysema.
f) The incidence of bronchiectasis is significantly reduced by corticosteroids.
g) Corticosteroids reduce bronchial inflammation.
h) Caseous tissue is reduced by corticosteroids.
i) Surgical excision is the best treatment for caseous lymph nodes.

Unit 11 Process 4 Method

Section 1   Presentation

1. Look and read:

Technique of mouth-to-mouth resuscitation

The patient should be placed on his back on a firm surface.

1 The operator should quickly clear out food, etc. from the mouth and throat 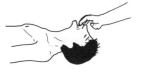 to prevent obstruction of the air passages.	2 The patient's head must be extended as far as possible 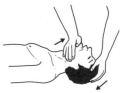 to ensure that the airway is kept open.
3 The operator should pinch the patient's nose with his fingers 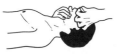 to prevent any leakage.	4 The operator's mouth should be sealed around the patient's mouth 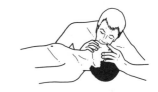 so that no air escapes.
5 Air is then blown into the lungs 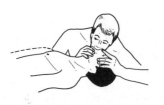 until the chest is seen to expand.	6 The operator should then remove his mouth quickly 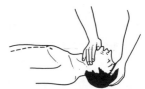 in order to allow passive expiration.

The process is repeated 10–15 times per minute (for an adult) until the patient's breathing begins again.

Now ask and answer questions like these:

Q {
What is the purpose of clearing out mucus, food, etc. from the mouth and throat?
Why should any mucus, food, etc. be cleared out from the mouth and throat?
}

A {
The purpose of clearing it out is to prevent obstruction.
To prevent obstruction of the air passages.
}

2. Read this example:

How is obstruction prevented?
Obstruction is prevented *by* clear*ing* the mouth and throat of mucus, food and other materials.

Answer these questions:

a) How is the airway kept open?
b) How are air leakages prevented?
c) How is expiration allowed to take place?
d) How does the operator extend the patient's head as far as possible?
e) How does the operator close the patient's nose?

3. You are supervising a demonstration of mouth-to-mouth resuscitation. Give instructions to the operator(s), beginning as follows:

'First *place* the patient on his back on a firm surface. Then ....'

Section 2   Development

4. Read this:

The physical examination of the abdomen: palpation

The examiner should stand, sit or kneel comfortably beside the patient. His hands should be warm. Palpation is undertaken in three phases: light palpation, deep palpation and bimanual palpation.

5   Light palpation should commence in an area removed from the site of any pain and the patient's face should be watched for any indication of tenderness or pain.

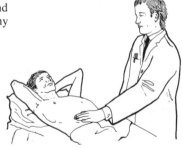

Complete/answer these:

a) To discover exactly where the pain is located, the examiner should ....
b) To enable him to carry out the examination properly, ...

c) Why should the examiner's hands be warm? (so that ......)
d) Why should palpation begin in an area where there is no pain? (so that ......)

Continue reading:

Muscle tone is tested by gentle dipping movements as the hand is moved from region to region without breaking contact with the skin. Localised rigidity is
10 usually associated with organic disease. Generalised rigidity commonly implies failure of the patient to relax but is also a feature of peritonitis when it is accompanied by tenderness. To test for this, the hand should be applied firmly and then suddenly removed: 'rebound pain' will indicate peritonitis.

(**Note:** 'rebound pain' refers to pain which is felt not from the pressure of the hand but when the hand is released.)

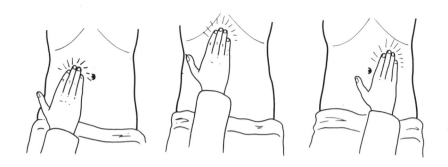

Testing muscle tone

Look at this example:

What is the significance of rebound pain?
Rebound pain *indicates* peritonitis.

e) What is the significance of rigidity in one part of the abdomen?
f) What is the significance of rigidity all over the abdomen plus slight pain on palpation?
g) What is the more likely significance of generalised rigidity alone?
h) What is the purpose of the gentle dipping movements?
i) How does the examiner test for peritonitis?
j) Demonstrate the technique of testing for muscle tone on a flat surface.

5. Read this:

Diagnosis of tuberculosis: the tuberculin test
With the *Mantoux* technique a solution of old tuberculin or purified protein derivative (PPD) tuberculin is injected intradermally on the anterior aspect of the forearm. The test should first be carried out with 1 tuberculin unit (TU) in 0·1 ml of normal saline. Often there will be no reaction, in which case the test
5 should be repeated with 10 TU in the same volume of saline. In order to obtain accurate results it is essential to use freshly prepared dilutions of tuberculin.

Complete these notes:

> Mantoux test
> 1 Injection of ...... tuberculin in ...... into ....
> 2 If no ......, further ...... of ....

(**Note:** tuberculin dilutions must ...... so that ....)

Sentences (a) to (g) describe another test. Rearrange them to follow this pattern:

> Introduction: Purpose of test
> Technique of test
> Findings/Results of test
> Significance of findings   (diagnosis)
> Treatment indicated

a) For this test a solution containing 100,000 TU of PPD tuberculin per ml normal saline, to which adrenaline has been added, should be used.
b) Four grades of positivity can be recognised, according to the severity of the skin reaction.
c) When large numbers of people (particularly children) are being tested for tuberculosis the *Heaf multiple puncture tuberculin test* is preferable to the Mantoux technique as it is more rapidly performed and is less painful.
d) All newly diagnosed patients should be treated with a combination of three drugs until further tests on the drug sensitivity of the tubercle bacillus can be completed.
e) The test may be read from the third to the seventh day.
f) A drop of testing fluid is placed on the skin of the forearm. The skin is tensed with the left hand and is then punctured to a depth of 2 mm using an instrument consisting of six short steel needles held in the right hand.
g) Reaction in grades III and IV indicates infection with mammalian tubercle bacilli.

6. Read this:

In the case of / When there is { diagnosis / symptom / disease } X, treatment Y *is indicated.*

Example: In the case of a diagnosis of tuberculosis, immediate commencement of chemotherapy *is indicated* using a combination of three drugs.

Now read this:

Symptomatic treatment of tuberculosis
Haemoptysis nearly always stops spontaneously, but a sedative may be given to allay anxiety, e.g. diazepam 5–10 mg, thrice daily. If the haemorrhage is very severe a blood transfusion should be given and, if respiratory obstruction develops, the blood must be removed from the bronchi by aspiration through a bronchoscope.

Answer these questions:

a) Three forms of treatment are described. What are they?
b) When is the transfusion of blood indicated?
c) When is aspiration of the blood from the lungs indicated?

d) Of the three methods of treatment, one is absolutely vital, or essential (i.e. without it the patient would probably die); another is important but not a matter of life and death; while the other is an optional one which is not important physically. Identify each.

e) Explain the difference in the severity of the three grades·of this condition by saying what you think would happen in each case if it were left untreated.

Section 3   Reading

7. Read this:

Symptomatic treatment in respiratory disease

Cough, when productive of sputum, should be encouraged and not suppressed. Those who are physically weak should be exhorted at regular intervals to clear their bronchi of secretion. Those with bronchiectasis or lung abscess should practise postural drainage, and those with tenacious sputum should be given hot
5 drinks and inhalations of either steam or nebulised water to help them to bring it up more easily.

Unproductive, distressing cough should be suppressed. Demulcent lozenges are occasionally effective, but many patients require antitussive drugs, especially if sleep is disturbed by coughing.

Airway obstruction in bronchitis and asthma is treated by bronchodilator
10 drugs and in certain carefully selected cases by corticosteroids.

Chest pain. Pleural pain can usually be relieved by the application of a rubber hot-water bottle or an electric heating pad to the chest wall, supplemented by an analgesic and, if necessary, by an antitussive drug. Mild analgesics, such as acetylsalicylic acid, or codeine compound tablets, are adequate in most cases
15 but a few patients may require pethidine, 50–100 mg by mouth or intramuscular injection, or even morphine, 10–15 mg subcutaneously. Opiates must, however, be avoided in patients with poor respiratory function and in those who have difficulty in coughing up sputum.

The pain of acute tracheitis usually responds to the application of heat to the
20 front of the chest, combined with inhalations of steam medicated with benzoin. Pain due to invasion of the chest wall by a malignant tumour, if not relieved by radiotherapy, usually demands a powerful analgesic such as pethidine or morphine, given by injection. In advanced cases these drugs may become ineffective and neurosurgical measures may be required for the relief of intractable
25 pain.

Summarise the passage by extending and completing this table:

INDICATIONS	TREATMENT	PURPOSE	
bronchiectasis; lung abscess	postural drainage	to clear bronchi	
tenacious sputum		} to suppress cough	

Answer these questions:

    a) When is the use of antitussive drugs indicated?
    b) How do bronchodilator drugs help to clear airway obstruction?
    c) When is the use of pethidine or morphine indicated?
    d) What is pethidine? How should it be administered?
    e) When is the use of morphine contraindicated? What do you think is the reason?
    f) How many methods of administering drugs are mentioned? Describe them.
    g) How many kinds of chest pain are mentioned? What are they?

Complete these sentences:

    h) If a patient is suffering from ......, he ...... postural drainage to ....
    i) In cases where ......, the patient can be helped ...... by ...... hot drinks and ....
    j) Demulcent lozenges are used ...... when there is ...... and the patient feels ......, although in cases where ...... these will often be inadequate and ....

8. Read this passage and give it a title:

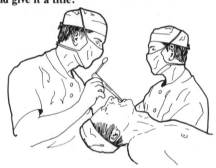

Bronchoscopy

Bronchoscopy is a relatively simple technique which involves passing a hollow tube down along the trachea in order to inspect the bronchi and remove foreign matter from them if necessary. Obviously a general or a local anaesthetic is required for this. The general preference seems to be for the former. Further-
5 more general anaesthesia permits a leisurely inspection of all the bronchial orifices, the aspiration of secretions, and the inflation of the affected lobe or lung.

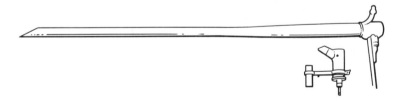

Bronchoscope of Negus type

    The instrument should be passed with great care and without force. Care must be taken to avoid tears distally and damage to the teeth proximally. The
10 bronchoscope must be removed immediately from a struggling patient.

Forceps and suckers can be passed down the inside of the bronchoscope to remove foreign bodies or aspirate foreign matter such as soft, caseous vegetable material. While performing this operation every attempt must be made to keep the field clear of blood by suction and to avoid impacting a foreign body
15 more deeply.

Bronchoscopy is indicated in a number of conditions. In carcinoma of the bronchus, for example, bronchoscopy is an essential diagnostic procedure. In any suspected case of an intrabronchial foreign body bronchoscopy must be performed both to confirm the diagnosis and, if possible, to withdraw the object.
20 And in cases where a benign tumour has been removed, bronchoscopy is advisable at regular intervals to detect a recurrence.

Indicate where to insert the following at appropriate points in the passage:

a) Moreover, if the lesion is centrally placed, the examination will show the presence of the tumour and enable a biopsy to be made.
b) In cases where inspection indicates the necessity
c) otherwise there is the risk of rupture of the air passages and possibly asphyxia.
d) as it is difficult to administer adequate local anaesthesia if there are excessive secretions in the pharynx and air passages.
e) Prolonged attempts at removal should not, however, be made owing to the risks of oedema of the glottis or of damaging the bronchial tree further.

9. Make notes on the passage. Then, at a later date, write a summary of the passage using only your notes.

Section 4　Listening

10. Listen to the passage which will be read to you, and make notes on it as it is being read, as if you were attending a lecture. You will find these headings and diagrams useful:

Aspiration of fluid from pleural space.
Purpose 1.
2.

Procedure/Technique
1. General
2.
3.

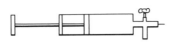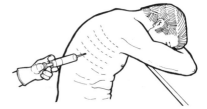

Use your notes as a guide to write a passage about aspirating fluid from the pleural space, but this time arrange the material as follows:

> General description
> Purpose 1: Indications, Procedure, Results
> Purpose 2: Indications, Procedure, Results
> Contraindications

Listen to the passage again to help you fill in any parts which are not sufficiently clear from your notes, and if there is anything which is not in your notes, nor in the passage, you will have to provide it yourself from your own medical knowledge.

Unit 12 Consolidation

1. Look at this table:

PROTOZOA	BACTERIA
Unicellular microorganisms	Unicellular microorganisms
2–100 μm	0·5–10 μm
Motile (e.g. amoeboid movement)	Usually nonmotile

Cell structure similar to animals'
– true nucleus (with surrounding
  membrane)
	Cell structure between animals' and
	  plants'
	– nuclear material, no membrane, no
	  nucleoli

Intracellular digestion (phagocytic)	Enzymatic activity at cell surface
Parasitic (a few to man)	Many parasitic

Reproduction:
  binary *and* multiple fission; many
  have complex life cycle, e.g. as
  trophozoite (active, feeding stage)
  and cyst (inactive stage)
	Reproduction:
	  binary fission

Sometimes antigenic	Antigenic
(i.e. produce formation of specific antibodies)	
Often pathogenic	Occasionally pathogenic

Can resist high concentrations of
  antibiotics
	Not resistant to high concentrations
	  of antibiotics

a) Compare protozoa and bacteria, using the following words and patterns:
    both ...... and ...... ; but; whereas; however; on the other hand;
    While protozoa are ......, bacteria are ....
    In protozoa, digestion takes place ...... while in bacteria ....
b) Write a description of protozoa.
c) Write a description of bacteria.

2. Read the passage and label the four diagrams referred to in the text:

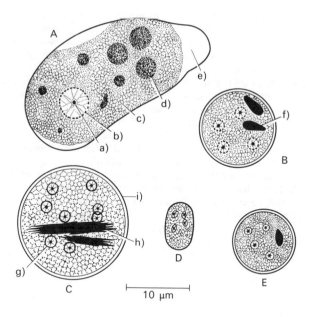

One of the main groups of protozoa is that consisting of the amoebae, eight species of which may infect man. These organisms vary in size, with species or stage of development, from some 5 to 50 µm in diameter; most are between 7 and 35 µm. Differentiation of species both as trophozoites and cysts tends to be
5 difficult: this depends on the size and details of nuclear structure and cytoplasmic inclusions, which are difficult to observe.

Only one species, *Entamoeba histolytica*, is regarded as an important pathogen. The trophozoite measures 20 to 40 µm in diameter and is made up of two kinds of cytoplasm: the clear, glasslike ectoplasm and the finely granulated
10 endoplasm in which the single nucleus is located and which contains ingested substances such as erythrocytes. This vegetative form is highly active and divides by binary fission. The cyst form of *E. histolytica* is less than half the diameter of the trophozoite and is spherical with a smooth wall and is translucent. Cysts contain one, two or four, but never more than four, nuclei. Thick ovoid or rod-
15 shaped structures known as chromatoid bodies may also be seen.

The character of the nuclei should be noted, particularly the ring of fine chromatin granules round the inner face of the nuclear membrane, and the small karyosome which is situated centrally. These features allow differentiation from the commensal *E. coli* where the karyosome is not centrally situated and the
20 chromatin is coarser.

E. histolytica was previously classified according to whether cysts were more or less than 10 µm diameter. It has been demonstrated, however, that cysts with a diameter of less than 10 µm are not pathogenic for human beings and are therefore now considered to be a different species, *E. hartmanni*, which is re-
25 garded as nonpathogenic.

    j) Write short descriptions of – the structure of an *E. coli* cyst.
                                  – properties of an *E. histolytica* trophozoite.
                                  – nuclear structure of *E. histolytica*.
    k) Compare the cyst and trophozoite forms of *E. histolytica*.

3. Read this passage and label the diagram on page 113:

Amoebiasis

The primary site of development of the pathogen *E. histolytica* is the lumen of the large intestine, where the amoebae may thrive, feeding on bacteria and re-producing by binary fission. This is the condition known as 'amoebiasis'. Often, and for reasons unknown, the amoebae penetrate the epithelium and multiply
5   in the gut wall causing ulceration and necrosis. From there they may spread to other tissues such as liver, lung and brain; infection of the liver with abscess formation is common, but abscesses in other sites are rare. In unfavourable conditions amoebae encyst; the cysts pass in the faeces and may remain viable and infective for several weeks outside the host. When cysts are ingested in water
10   or food, they pass unaltered through the stomach and become activated in the small intestine. The cytoplasm starts to stream and the amoeba squeezes through a small hole in the cyst wall and escapes (excystation).

    The trophozoites which emerge from the cysts colonise the large intestine and may live in the lumen for long periods without invading the tissues. In such cases
15   *E. histolytica* will be excreted in the faeces (after encystation), often in large numbers, although there are no signs of intestinal disturbance. Under certain conditions, however, invasion and ulceration of the mucous membrane of the large bowel takes place resulting in symptoms of amoebic dysentery. The lesions are usually maximal in the caecum although as the condition develops further
20   lesions may be produced, particularly in the sigmoid colon and rectum. From the primary site in the intestine amoebae may find their way into a vein and be carried to the liver where they multiply and cause hepatocellular necrosis ('amoebic abscess').

    Rarely the amoebic ulcers penetrate through the muscular coat of the colon,
25   perforating the peritoneum. Normally, however, they spread only within the submucosa, and although the lesions on the surface of the mucosa are usually small (with raised edges) they overlie larger widening areas of necrosis in the submucosa, producing bottle-shaped lesions. The development of these ulcers follows an initial stage of abscess formation after the invasion of the mucosa
30   by trophozoites and their penetration into the submucosa. Once there, they multiply to form the abscess which subsequently ruptures into the lumen forming the ulcer. Cysts are not found amongst amoebae growing in the tissues. To complete the life cycle, conditions must be favourable both for growth and for cyst formation.
35   On being excreted in the faeces, cysts may infect other hosts in a number of ways. The faeces may directly contaminate water, which is then drunk; insects such as flies may transfer cysts from faeces to food; or the cysts may be trans-mitted by a (human) food-handler. Ingestion of trophozoites, on the other hand, is not infectious because they are not resistant to the digestive action of gastric
40   juices.

a) Describe the life cycle of *E. histolytica*, beginning with its ingestion by a host.
b) What is the difference between 'amoebiasis' and 'amoebic dysentery'?
c) Describe a symptomless case of amoebiasis.
d) Describe the process of ulcer formation.
e) Why do trophozoites usually encyst before being excreted?

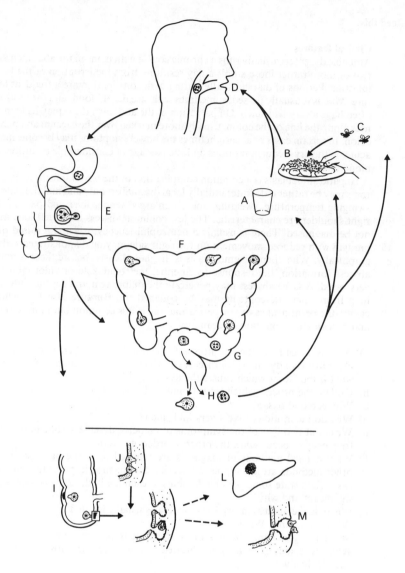

The spread of amoebiasis and some developments

f) Why do the amoebae invade the mucosal membrane of the colon?
g) What are the effects of this?
h) How are the amoebae carried to the liver?
i) What are the effects of this?
j) Where are ulcers most often found in amoebic dysentery?
k) What are the chances of a perforated peritoneum developing from amoebiasis?
l) What happens to *E. histolytica* in the stomach?

4. Read this:

Clinical features

Amoebic dysentery usually runs a chronic course with pains in the abdomen and two or more rather loose stools a day resulting from the irritation of the large intestine. Periods of diarrhoea alternating with constipation are a frequent feature. Mucus is usually passed, sometimes with streaks of blood, and the motions
5 often have a very bad smell. On palpation of the abdomen there may be tenderness along the line of the colon, usually more marked over the caecum and pelvic colon. In certain cases or at certain times the bowel symptoms may become more acute, with very frequent motions and the passage of considerable quantities of blood and mucus.
10 Hepatic amoebiasis is a common complication of the bowel infection. Symptoms may be rather indefinite: initially local discomfort only and malaise; later a swinging temperature, sweating, and an enlarged tender liver and pain in the right shoulder are characteristic. The less common abscess in the left lobe may not be diagnosed. There is usually a neutrophil leucocytosis and a raised dia-
15 phragm with reduced movement on the right side may be demonstrated radiographically. When hepatic amoebiasis is diagnosed early, before there is much abscess formation, the response to emetine, metronidazole or chloroquine is very rapid. A large abscess may penetrate the diaphragm and rupture into the lung from where its contents may be coughed up. Rupture into the pleural
20 cavity, the peritoneal cavity or pericardial sac is less common but more serious and necessitates aspiration or drainage.

a) What is the cause of the symptoms of amoebic dysentery? Do you know any other forms of dysentery, or diseases in which dysentery occurs? In each case what is the factor which causes the dysentery?
b) Explain the process which leads to mucus being passed.
c) Why is blood passed?
d) Why do the motions have a very bad smell?
e) Write out two lists of the symptoms of amoebic dysentery: one in order of frequency of occurrence, the other in order of severity.
f) What clinical methods of diagnosis are referred to in the passage? What other methods are mentioned? Describe the diagnostic procedure in each case. Then state some possible findings of each method, say which ones are significant and why.
g) Where is the abscess in hepatic amoebiasis usually located?
h) What is emetine? What is its effect?
i) In what way can amoebic dysentery affect the respiratory system?
j) What treatment or therapy is indicated in cases where the abscess ruptures outside the liver?

5. Listen to the passage about the diagnosis of amoebiasis and make notes about the diagnostic procedures which are used (including any special instructions) and their purposes:

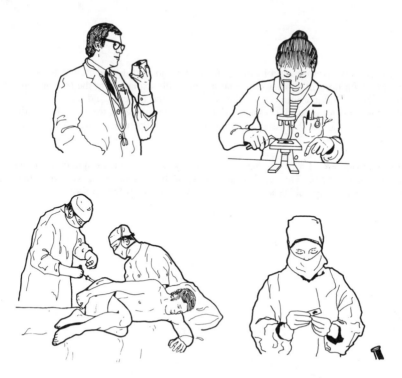

Identify the diagrams and write your notes under the headings below.

Diagnosis of amoebiasis	
(PROCEDURE)	(PURPOSE)

Glossary

This list gives the pronunciations of the technical and semi-technical words used in this book and definitions of those words that are not fully explained in the text or diagrams. It also includes some common word-elements (prefixes, stems and suffixes) which are used in biology. An asterisk (*) means that a word in the definition is itself explained in the Glossary. The number after each entry indicates the unit in which the word first appears.

Pronunciations are shown in the system that is used in the Longman *Dictionary of Contemporary English*. The symbols are shown in this table, with a key word for each. The letters printed in **bold type** represent the sound value of the symbol.

Consonants

p	**p**ea	f	**f**ew	ʃ	**fish**ing	h	**h**ot
b	**b**ay	v	**v**iew	ʒ	plea**s**ure	m	su**m**
t	**t**ea	θ	**th**ing	tʃ	**ch**oose	n	su**n**
d	**d**ay	ð	**th**en	dʒ	**j**ump	ŋ	su**ng**
k	**k**ey	s	**s**oon	l	**l**ed	j	**y**et
g	**g**ay	z	**z**oo	r	**r**ed	w	**w**et

Vowels

iː	sh**ee**p	ɔː	c**augh**t	eɪ	m**a**ke	ɪə	h**ere**
ɪ	sh**i**p	ʊ	p**u**t	əʊ	n**o**te	eə	th**ere**
e	b**e**d	uː	b**oo**t	aɪ	b**i**te	ʊə	p**oor**
æ	b**a**d	ʌ	c**u**t	aʊ	n**ow**	eɪə	pl**ayer**
ɑː	c**al**m	ɜː	b**ir**d	ɔɪ	b**oy**	əʊə	l**ower**
ɒ	c**o**t	ə	**a**bout			aɪə	t**ire**
						aʊə	t**ower**
						ɔɪə	empl**oyer**

Notes

1. A small raised /ʳ/ at the end of a word means that the /r/ is pronounced if a vowel follows (at the beginning of the next word), but not otherwise. For example, *far* /fɑːʳ/ means that *far away* is pronounced /fɑːr əweɪ/ but *far down* is /fɑː daʊn/.

2. The italic /ə/ means that the sound /ə/ can be used but is often omitted. It may be found before the consonants /m, n, ŋ, l, r/ in certain positions. For example, *travel* /ˈtrævəl/ means that the pronunciation /ˈtrævəl/ is possible but /ˈtrævl/ may be more common.

3. The mark /ˈ/ means that the following syllable has *main stress*, and /ˌ/ means that the following syllable has *secondary stress*. For example, *understand* /ˌʌndəˈstænd/.

a-; an- without, reduced level of (anoxia*)

abdomen /ˈæbdəmən/; **abdominal** (*adj.*) /æbˈdɒmɪnəl/ 2

abscess /ˈæbses/ a collection of pus* resulting from infection* by bacteria 11

absorb /əbˈzɔːb, -ˈsɔːb/ to take in by chemical or molecular action B

acetoacetic acid /əˌsiːtəʊəˈsiːtɪk ˈæsɪd/ 9

acetylsalicylic acid /əˌsiːtaɪlˌsælɪˈsɪlɪk/ aspirin, an analgesic* drug 11

ache /eɪk/ a constant pain 10

acid /ˈæsɪd/; **acidosis** /æsɪˈdəʊsɪs/ 9

activate /ˈæktɪveɪt/ to stimulate* 5

acute /əˈkjuːt/ sharp, severe; having a quick start, short course and severe symptoms* 10

adhesive /ədˈhiːsɪv/ 1

adipose /ˈædɪpəʊs/ fatty, fat-like 3

adrenalin(e) /əˈdrenəlɪn/ a hormone* produced by the adrenal /əˈdriːnəl/ or suprarenal gland 11

-aem (see haem)

aetiology /ˌiːtɪˈɒlədʒɪ/ the study of causes of disease 10

afferent /ˈæfərənt/ carrying towards B

alimentary canal /ælɪˌmentərɪ kəˈnæl/ 2

alkali /ˈælkəlaɪ/; **alkaline** (*adj.*) /-laɪn/ 9

allergy /ˈælədʒɪ/ the production of antibodies against harmless factors 10

alveolus /ælˈviːələs, ælvɪˈəʊləs/ *pl.* **alveoli** /-aɪ/ small cavity or air cell in the lung 7

amino (acid) /əˈmaɪnəʊ, əˈmiːnəʊ/ 5

amoeba /əˈmiːbə/ *pl.* **amoebae** /-biː/ 1

amoebiasis /ˌæmiːˈbaɪəsɪs/ infection* with *E. histolytica* 12

anaemia /əˈniːmɪə/ shortage of haemoglobin in the blood 6

anaesthesia /ˌænəsˈθiːzɪə/ the state of being unable to feel (pain, heat, etc.) 11

anaesthetic /ˌænəsˈθetɪk/ a substance that produces anaesthesia* 11

analgesic /ˌænəlˈdʒiːzɪk/ a pain-relieving drug 11

anatomy /əˈnætəmɪ/ the study of the structure of the body and its organs 2

angular notch /ˌæŋɡjʊlə ˈnɒtʃ/ 2

ankle /ˈæŋkəl/ 2

anorexia /ˌænəˈreksɪə/ loss of appetite 8

anoxia /æˈnɒksɪə/ 7

anti- against

antibiotic /ˌæntɪbaɪˈɒtɪk/ a product of one organism* used against infections* caused by other organisms 12

antibody /ˈæntɪbɒdɪ/ 5

antigen /ˈæntɪdʒən/ a foreign substance against which the body forms an antibody 5

antitussive /ˌæntɪˈtʌsɪv/ cough relieving 11

antrum /ˈæntrəm/ 2

anxiety /æŋˈzaɪətɪ/ a feeling of fear or uncertainty 4

aorta /eɪˈɔːtə/ 2

appendix /əˈpendɪks/ 2

aqueous humor /ˌeɪkwiːəs ˈhjuːmə, ækw-/ 3

artery /ˈɑːtərɪ/ any vessel carrying blood away from the heart 1

arteriole /ɑːˈtɪərɪəʊl/ a small twig of an artery* leading to capillaries 1

artificial /ɑːtɪˈfɪʃəl/ not natural, man-made, not real 5

ascorbate /æsˈkɔːbeɪt/ a salt of ascorbic acid (vitamin C) 7

asphyxia /æsˈfɪksɪə/ 7

aspirate /ˈæspɪreɪt/ to withdraw or remove a gas or fluid from a cavity, vessel, or enclosed space by suction 11

asthma /ˈæsmə/ a respiratory disease in which breathing is made difficult because of contraction of the muscles surrounding the bronchi* 11

axilla /ækˈsɪlə/ the armpit; the space between the upper part of the arm and the side wall of the chest; **axillary** (*adj.*) /ækˈsɪlərɪ/ 4

bacillus /bəˈsɪləs/ *pl.* **bacilli** /-laɪ/ 1

Bacillus megaterium /bəˌsɪləs megəˈtɪərɪəm/ 1

bacterium /bækˈtɪərɪəm/ *pl.* **bacteria** /-rɪə/ 1

basal /ˈbeɪsəl/ (of metabolism*) the resting rate of C

base /beɪs/ a substance capable of combining with an acid to form a neutral salt (cf. alkali*) 9

benign /bəˈnaɪn/ (of a tumour*) not dangerous, not malignant* 11

benzoin /ˈbenzəʊɪn/ an analgesic* 11

bi- two

bicarbonate /baɪˈkɑːbəneɪt/ HCO_3 9

bile /baɪl/ a thick, yellow-brown fluid secreted by the liver 2

binary /ˈbaɪnərɪ/ divided or dividing in two 12

bio- life; relating to living organisms*

biology /baɪˈɒlədʒɪ/ the science or study of life 5

biopsy /ˈbaɪɒpsɪ/ the removal and

examination of living tissue for diagnostic purposes 11

blastocyst /'blæstəsɪst/ a spherical mass containing a cavity surrounded by a layer of cells; early stage of an embryo* 6

bond /bɒnd/ the joining force between adjacent atoms 7

bowel /'baʊəl/ the intestine 10

breed /briːd/ to reproduce* 6

bronchiectasis /ˌbrɒŋkɪ'ektəsɪs/ a chronic dilatation* of the bronchi* in which they cannot clear secretions 10

bronchiole /'brɒŋkɪəʊl/ a very small branch of a bronchus* 3

bronchitis /brɒŋ'kaɪtəs/ inflammation* of the air passages in the lungs 10

bronchoscope /'brɒŋkəskəʊp/ 11

bronchoscopy /ˌbrɒŋ'kɒskəpɪ/ 11

bronchus /'brɒŋkəs/ pl. **bronchi** /-kaɪ/ air passage in the lung 4

buccal /'bʌkəl/ of the cheek 4

bud /bʌd/ undeveloped form of an organ or a part of the body 6

buffer /'bʌfə^r/ to reduce a change in pH 9

cadaver /kə'dævə^r/ a dead body 4

caecum /'siːkəm/ pl. **caeca** /-kə/ 2

calcify /'kælsɪfaɪ/ to deposit or lay down calcium salts 10

calculus /'kælkjʊləs/ a stone in part of the body; pl. **calculi** /-laɪ/ 10

calyx /'kælɪks/ pl. **calyces** /'kælɪsiːs/ A

cancer /'kænsə/ (a disease involving) a malignant* tumour* 4

capillary /kə'pɪlərɪ/ 1

capsule /'kæpsjuːl/ A

carbohydrate /ˌkɑːbəʊ'haɪdreɪt/ a compound of carbon, hydrogen, and oxygen (e.g. sugars and starches) 7

carcinoma /ˌkɑːsɪ'nəʊmə/ a cancer* 11

cardiac /'kɑːdɪæk/ of the heart 2

caseous /'keɪsɪəs/ of or like cheese; (of dying tissue which looks) like cheese 10

catabolism /kæ'tæbəlɪzəm/ the chemical breakdown in the body of complex substances to simple ones 8

caudal /'kɔːdəl/ 2

cercaria /sɜː'kærɪə/ pl. **-riae** /-riiː/ 6

cerebellum /serə'beləm/ 3

cerebrum /'serəbrəm/ 3

cervical /'sɜːvɪkəl/ of the neck (cervix) 2

characteristic /ˌkærəktə'rɪstɪk/ a symptom* which is typical of a disease; **characterise** (v.) /'kærəktəraɪz/ 8

chemotherapy /ˌkeməʊ'θerəpɪ/ treatment* with drugs 10

chest /tʃest/ thorax 10

chloroquine /'klɔːrəkwiːn,-ɪn/ 12

cholesterol /kə'lestərɒl/ 12

choroid /'kɒrɔɪd/ 3

chromatin /'krəʊmətɪn/ 3

ciliary /'sɪlɪərɪ/ 3

citrus fruits /'sɪtrəs fruːts/ the group of fruits including oranges, lemons, etc. 7

clavicle /'klævɪkəl/ 2

clinical /'klɪnɪkəl/ relating to bedside treatment* or the symptoms* and course of a disease 7

Clostridium sporogenes /klɒsˌtrɪdɪəm spɒ'rɒdʒiniːz/ 1

coccus /'kɒkəs/ pl. **cocci** /'kɒksaɪ/ 1

coccyx /'kɒksɪks/ 2

codeine /'kəʊdiːn/ an alkaloid drug (from opium) used to relieve pain and suppress cough 11

coil /kɔɪl/ a spiral 2

collagen /'kɒlədʒən/ a protein 3

colon /'kəʊlən/ 1

column /'kɒləm/ a long, thin, straight vertical structure (usually cylindrical in shape); **columnar** (adj.) /kə'lʌmnə^r/ 2

coma /'kəʊmə/ unconsciousness from which a patient cannot be woken 8

commensal /kə'mensəl/ a harmless parasite* 12

compartment /kəm'pɑːtmənt/ a division of an enclosed space 3

compensatory /ˌkɒmpən'seɪtərɪ/ making up for a loss 8

complication /ˌkɒmplɪ'keɪʃən/ a second condition or disease occurring in the course of a first 10

concave /'kɒnkeɪv/ with a surface curved like the inside of a circle or sphere 1

concentrate /'kɒnsəntreɪt/ to make a solution stronger 5

congenital /kən'dʒenɪtl/ present from or before birth 10

conjunctiva /ˌkɒndʒʌŋk'taɪvə/ 3

connective tissue /kəˌnektɪv 'tɪʃuː/ the material which separates, protects and supports the organs* 3

conscious /'kɒnʃəs/ mentally awake and aware 8

contaminate /kən'tæmɪneɪt/ to bring (harmful) bacteria into contact with; to infect* 12

contract /kən'trækt/ to draw the parts together; to become smaller 5

convex /'kɒnveks/ with a surface curved like the outside of a circle or sphere 1

convoluted /ˌkɒnvə'luːtɪd/ folded in

curves; coiled A

cornea /'kɔːnɪə/ 3

coronal /kə'rəʊnəl/ 2

cortex /'kɔːtɛks/ outer layer of an organ* A

corticosteroids /ˌkɔːtɪkəʊ'stɪərɔɪdz/ steroids having properties like those of the hormones* of the adrenal cortex 9

cough /kɒf/ a sudden, violent, noisy expulsion of air from the lungs 10

cranium /'kreɪnɪəm/ bones of the head; skull; **cranial** (adj.) /'kreɪnɪəl/ 2

curvature /'kɜːvətʃəʳ/ (amount of) curving or bending 1

cutaneous /kjʊ'teɪnɪəs/ of the skin (cutis) 3

cyanide /'saɪənaɪd/ a quick-acting poison* 7

cyanosis /ˌsaɪə'nəʊsɪs/ a condition in which parts of the body turn blue from lack of oxygen 10

cycle /'saɪkəl/ a process which continuously repeats itself 6

cylinder /'sɪlɪndə/; **cylindrical** (adj.) /sɪ'lɪndrɪkəl/ 1

cyst /sɪst/ 12

-cyte cell (e.g. leucocyte)

cytoplasm /'saɪtəʊplæzəm/ 3

damage /'dæmɪdʒ/ harm, injury* 8

dehydration /ˌdiːhaɪ'dreɪʃən/ the removal of water (from the body or tissues) C

demulcent /dɪ'mʌlsənt/ soothing; relieving irritation* of surfaces 11

depress /dɪ'pres/ to decrease the normal activity of 9

deplete /dɪ'pliːt/ to reduce the quantity (of stored materials) 7

deprivation /ˌdeprɪ'veɪʃən/ a condition of being in want of a certain thing 7

derived /dɪ'raɪvd/ formed or developed from something else 3

dermis /'dɜːmɪs/ 3

destroy /dɪ'strɔɪ/ to cause the death of; to break up; **destruction** (n.) /dɪ'strʌkʃən/ 5

diabetes mellitus /daɪəˌbiːtiːz 'melɪtəs/ 7

diabetes insipidus /daɪəˌbiːtiːz ɪn'sɪpɪdəs/ C

diagnosis /ˌdaɪəg'nəʊsɪs/ the identification or recognition of disease* 11

diaphragm /'daɪəfræm/ 1

diarrhoea /ˌdaɪə'rɪə/ the frequent passage of watery stools* 7

diastolic /ˌdaɪə'stɒlɪk/ of the phase of relaxation of the heart muscle 4

diazepam /daɪ'æzəpæm, daɪ'eɪzəpæm/ 11

diet /'daɪət/ the sort of food usually eaten by a person, community, etc. 10

differentiate /ˌdɪfə'renʃɪeɪt/ to see or recognise the difference between 12

digestion /daɪ'dʒestʃən/ the process of converting food into a form in which it can be absorbed*; **di'gest** (v.); **di'gestive** (adj.) 5

diguanide /daɪ'gwænaɪd/ 8

dilate /daɪ'leɪt, dɪ'l-/ to enlarge or stretch; **dilatation** (n.) /dɪlə'teɪʃən/ or **dilation** /daɪ'leɪʃən/ 1

dilute /daɪ'luːt/ to reduce the strength of a solution 11

Diplococcus pneumoniae /dɪpləˌkɒkəs njuː'məʊnɪaɪ/ 1

-dips(o)- thirst*

discharge /dɪs'tʃɑːdʒ/ to release or to let something go 10

disease /dɪ'ziːz/ an illness or sickness 5

disseminate /dɪ'semɪneɪt/ to distribute* widely 10

distal /'dɪstəl/ 2

distribute /dɪs'trɪbjuːt/ to spread around, send to different points 5

disturbance /dɪs'tɜːbəns/ a harmful change in function or structure; **disturb** (v.) /dɪs'tɜːb/

diuresis /daɪjʊ'riːsɪs/ an artificially increased flow of urine 8

diuretic /ˌdaɪjʊ'retɪk/ a substance which increases the flow of urine 8

dorsal /'dɔːsəl/ of the back 2

dosage /'dəʊsɪdʒ/ size of dose* 4

dose /dəʊs/ the amount of medicine (drug) to be taken at one time 4

drainage /'dreɪnɪdʒ/ the provision of a way of escape for fluid from a cavity 11

drowsy /'draʊzɪ/ sleepy 8

duct /dʌkt/ a tube for carrying fluids (secretions of glands or organs) A

duodenum /djuːə'diːnəm/ 1

dys- (dis-) bad; difficult

dysentery /'dɪsəntrɪ/ inflammation* of the large intestine causing diarrhoea* with blood, mucus*, pain and fever 6

dysuria /dɪs'jʊrɪə/ difficulty or pain in urination 10

ect(o)- outside, outer

ectoderm /'ektədɜːm/ the outer layer of cells in an embryo* from which skin and nervous system develop 3

-ectomy surgical removal of a part of the

body

efferent /'efərənt/ carrying away B

electrocardiograph /ɪˌlektrəʊ'kɑːdɪəgræf/ 5

ellipsoid /ɪ'lɪpsɔɪd/ a (roughly) oval-shaped solid 1

elongate /'iːlɒŋgeɪt/ to make or become longer 1

embedded /em'bedəd/ firmly fixed in surrounding material 3

embryo /'embrɪəʊ/ the unborn child during the first 2 months in the uterus 6

embryonic /embrɪ'ɒnɪk/ in undeveloped form 3

emetine /'emətiːn, -ɪn/ 12

emotion /ɪ'məʊʃən/ a (strong) feeling 4

emphysema /ˌemfɪ'siːmə/ an abnormal presence of air in certain parts of the body 10

empyema /empaɪ'iːmə/ the presence of pus* in a cavity, hollow organ or body space 11

end(o)- within, inside, inner

endocrine glands /'endəʊkrɪn glændz/ glands which secrete their hormones* directly into the blood stream (internally) 4

endoderm /'endəd ɜːm/ the inner layer of cells in an embryo* from which the digestive organs and lungs develop 6

endoplasmic reticulum /endəˌplæzmɪk re'tɪkjələm/ 1

engulf /ɪn'gʌlf/ to swallow up; eat 5

Entamoeba /ˌentə'miːbə/; E. coli /-'kəʊlaɪ/; E. hartmanni /-'hɑːtmənaɪ/; E. histolytica /- hɪstəʊ'lɪtɪkə/ 12

enzyme /'enzaɪm/ a substance produced by living cells which stimulates chemical changes 5

epicardium /epɪ'kɑːdɪəm/ 3

epidemiology /ˌepɪdiːmɪ'ɒlədʒɪ/ the study of the occurrence and distribution* of diseases 6

epidermis /ˌepɪ'dɜːmɪs/ 3

epithelium /ˌepɪ'θiːlɪəm/ 3

erythrocyte /e'rɪθrəsaɪt/ 1

excrete /ɪks'kriːt/ to pass out unwanted products of metabolism* 5

exercise /'eksəsaɪz/ the use of muscles to improve health (e.g. by running) 9

expiration /ekspɪ'reɪʃən/ the act of breathing out 11

external /ɪks't ɜːnəl/ 2

eye /aɪ/ 1

faeces /'fiːsiːz/ the waste matter excreted*

from the intestines 6

fascia /'fæʃɪə/ thin, flat sheets of fibrous tissue under the skin and around muscles and other organs 3

fatigue /fə'tiːg/ tiredness 8

fever /'fiːvəʳ/ increased body temperature 8

fibre /'faɪbəʳ/ a long, thin strand of material which strengthens tissue or holds it together; fibrous (adj.) 3

fission /'fɪʃən/ division; asexual reproduction* 12

flatworm /'flætwɜːm/ one of a group of worms which includes tapeworms and flukes* 6

flexure /'flekʃəʳ/ a bend, curve or turn 2

fluid /'fluːɪd/ a liquid (or gas); not solid 5

fluke /fluːk/ a parasitic* worm which needs two hosts* 6

focus /'fəʊkəs/ the principal site* (of a disease) 10

foetus /'fiːtəs/ the unborn child from 3rd to 9th month in the uterus 5

forceps /'fɔːseps/ an instrument for taking hold of things 11

frequency /'friːkwənsɪ/ repeated urination after short intervals 10

fundus /'fʌndəs/ 2

gallbladder /'gɔːlblædəʳ/ 1

gastric /'gæstrɪk/ of the stomach 2

genetics /dʒə'netɪks/ the study of heredity and the physiology* of reproduction* 6

genital /'dʒenɪtl/ concerning (the organs of) reproduction* 4

germ /dʒɜːm/ an early stage in the development of an organism* 6

glomerulus /glɒ'merjʊləs/pl. glomeruli /-laɪ/ A

glottis /'glɒtɪs/ the narrow opening at the upper end of the larynx 11

glucose /'gluːkəʊs, -z/ a simple sugar 3

-glycaemia /-glaɪ'siːmɪə/

glycogen /'glaɪkəʊdʒən/ the main carbohydrate reserve, easily converted into glucose* 3

glycosuria /ˌglaɪkəʊ'sjʊərɪə/ 7

Golgi apparatus /ˌgɒldʒɪ æpə'reɪtəs/ 3

granule /'grænjuːl/ a very small (intra-cellular) particle* or mass 12

gut /gʌt/ the intestine 12

gynaecology /ˌgaɪnə'kɒlədʒɪ/ the medicine and surgery* of the female reproductive system 6

haem-, haemat(o)- blood

haematogenous /ˌhiːmə'tɒdʒənəs/ of

anything produced from, derived* from, or transported by the blood 10

haematopoiesis /hiːˌmætəʊpɔɪˈiːsɪs/ the proccss of formation and development of blood cells 4

haematuria /ˌhiːməˈtjʊərɪə/ blood in the urine 10

haemoptysis /hiːˈmɒptɪsɪs/ the spitting of blood from the lungs or bronchi* 11

haemorrhage /ˈhemərɪdʒ/ bleeding; the escape of blood from blood vessels 7

harm /hɑːm/ damage; injury* 5

healing /ˈhiːlɪŋ/ the process or act of getting well or making whole; the restoration of diseased parts; **heal** (v.) /hiːl/ 7

heart /hɑːt/ 1

helix /ˈhiːlɪks/ spiral; **helicoidal** (adj.) /ˌhelɪˈkɔɪdəl/ 1

hem-, hemato- (see **haem-, haemato-**)

Henle /ˈhenlɪ/ A

hepatic /hɪˈpætɪk/ of the liver 2

hereditary /həˈredɪtərɪ/ (of a disease) transmitted from parents to children 5

hilus /ˈhaɪləs/ A

hist(o)- tissue

histology /hɪsˈtɒlədʒɪ/ the study of the (minute structure of the) tissues 6

histotoxic /ˌhɪstəˈtɒksɪk/ poisonous* to the tissues 7

homeostasis /ˌhəʊmɪəʊˈsteɪsɪs, ˌhɒm-/ the process of maintaining constant physical and chemical conditions in the body; **homeostatic** (adj.) /ˌhəʊmɪəʊˈstætɪk/ C

hormone /ˈhɔːməʊn/ a substance released into the blood stream by one organ* to regulate the function of others 5

host /həʊst/ the organism* on which a parasite* lives 6

hydrochloric acid /ˌhaɪdrəˈklɔːrɪk ˈæsɪd/ HCl 9

-hydr(o)- water, hydrogen

β-hydroxybutyric /ˌbeɪtə haɪˌdrɒksɪbjuːˈtɪrɪk/ 8

hyper- excess of; above

hyperpnoea /haɪpəˈniːə/ 9

hyperglycaemia /ˌhaɪpəglaɪˈsiːmɪə/ 7

hyperplasia /ˌhaɪpəˈpleɪzɪə/ 7

hypertrophy /haɪˈpɜːtrəfɪ/ 7

hypo- lack of; under

hypothalamus /ˌhaɪpəʊˈθæləməs/ 9

-ia a condition, especially an abnormal or pathologic* condition

-ic of or related to

iliac /ˈɪlɪæk/ 2

immunity /ɪˈmjuːnɪtɪ/ natural resistance to infection* or disease 5

impact /ɪmˈpækt/ to pack or drive firmly together 11

in- (im-) not, non-, un-; in, into

incidence /ˈɪnsɪdəns/ the rate of occurrence (of a disease) 4

incubation /ˌɪŋkjʊˈbeɪʃən/ the period of time between infection* and the appearance of symptoms* 6

indicate /ˈɪndɪkeɪt/ to point to the cause, diagnosis*, treatment* or prognosis* of a disease* 8

infect /ɪnˈfekt/ to pass on a disease* or pathogenic* organism*; (of an organism*) to invade a body or organ*, to cause an infection* 6

infection /ɪnˈfekʃən/ the invasion of a host* by pathogenic* organisms*; the pathologic* state caused by organisms. 6

infectious /ɪnˈfekʃəs/ caused by infection; able to infect 6

inferior /ɪnˈfɪərɪə/ 2

inflammation /ˌɪnfləˈmeɪʃən/ the reaction to injury*, irritation* or infection*, involving redness, swelling, heat and pain 6

influenza /ˌɪnflʊˈenzə/ 10

ingest /ɪnˈdʒest/ to take food or other substances into the body (or into a cell) 5

inhale /ɪnˈheɪl/ to breathe in 7

inhalation /ɪnhəˈleɪʃən/ the process of inhaling; a drug taken by inhaling 11

inhibit /ɪnˈhɪbɪt/ to decrease or stop the normal action of an organ, cell or chemical 8

inject /ɪnˈdʒekt/ to put fluids into the skin, muscles, vessels or cavities 5

injury /ˈɪndʒərɪ/ the result of an action which changes the normal structure or function of an organ, with pathologic* effects 5

insulin /ˈɪnsjʊlɪn/ 7

intestine /ɪnˈtestɪn/ 1

intra- within, inside, into

intractable /ɪnˈtræktəbəl/ not easily managed or treated 11

ion /ˈaɪən/ an atom which has more or less than the normal number of electrons (and so conducts electricity) 9

iris /ˈaɪrɪs/ 3

irritate /'ɪrɪteɪt/ to alter or disturb* the normal function of an organ 12

isthmus /'ɪsməs/ 2

-itis inflammation* of a part

jejunum /dʒɪ'dʒuːnəm/ 2

joint /dʒɔɪnt/ the attachment between two bones 10

juice /dʒuːs/ the secretions of 12

karyosome /'kærɪəsəʊm/ 12

ketone /'kiːtəʊn/ 8

kidney /'kɪdnɪ/ 1

knee /niː/ 2

lactate /læk'teɪt/ to secrete milk 7

lactic acid /ˌlæktɪk 'æsɪd/ 9

larynx /'lærɪŋks/ 2

lateral /'lætərəl/ 2

lesion /'liːʒən/ a structural or functional change in an organ due to disease* (or injury) 10

leuc(o)-, leuko- white, (colourless)

leucocyte /'luːkəsaɪt/ 1

leucocytosis /ˌluːkəsaɪ'təʊsɪs/ 7

leucopenia /ˌluːkə'piːnɪə/ 7

limb /lɪm/ a long, thin structure, extending from the main part A

lipase /'laɪpeɪz/ an enzyme* which breaks down fat 5

lipid /'lɪpɪd/ a fat, or fat-like substance 3

lipolysis /lɪ'pɒlɪsɪs/ the dissolution of fat in water 8

liver /'lɪvəʳ/ 1

lobe /ləʊb/ a more or less rounded part of an organ, separated from other parts 2

local /'ləʊkəl/ limited to one part or place 12

longitudinal /ˌlɒndʒɪ'tjuːdənəl/ along the length (cf. sagittal or coronal sections) A

lozenge /'lɒzɪndʒ/ a soothing tablet or drug which is dissolved in the mouth 11

lumbar /'lʌmbəʳ/ of the back 2

lumen /'luːmən/ the space inside a tube B

lung /lʌŋ/ 1

lymph /lɪmf/ the part of the tissue fluid which is carried by special vessels (lymphatic vessels) 3

lymphosarcoma /ˌlɪmfəʊsɑː'kəʊmə/ a cancer* of the lymphatic tissues 10

-lysis dissolving, loosening, decomposition

lysosome /'laɪsəsəʊm/ 3

macr(o)- large, great; long

macrophage /'mækrəfeɪdʒ/ a large phagocytic cell (usually in the tissues) 5

macroscopic /ˌmækrə'skɒpɪk/ large enough to be seen by the naked eye 10

mal- wrong, abnormal, bad

malaise /mə'leɪz/ a general feeling of illness or discomfort 12

malignant /mə'lɪgnənt/ (of a tumour*) continuing to grow and spread, leading to death 11

mature /mə'tʊəʳ/ (adj.) fully developed, full grown; (v.) to become mature 5

maxillary sinus /mækˌsɪlərɪ 'saɪnəs/ an air-containing cavity in the upper jaw-bone, connected to the nose 10

mean /miːn/ the mid point between two extremes (maximum and minimum) 4

medial /'miːdɪəl/ 2

mediastinum /ˌmiːdɪəs'taɪnəm/ 3

medulla /mə'dʊlə/ bone marrow 3; the inner part of certain organs A

medulla oblongata /-ˌɒblɒŋ'gɑːtə/ 3

-megaly abnormal enlargement of

membrane /'membreɪn/ 3

meningism /'menɪndʒɪzm/ a condition with symptoms like those of meningitis* but due simply to a feverish state 10

meningitis /ˌmenɪn'dʒaɪtɪs/ inflammation* of the membranes of the brain or spinal cord 10

mesentery /'mezəntərɪ/ the part of the peritoneum* which attaches the intestines to the posterior abdominal wall; **mesenteric** (adj.) /mezən'terɪk/ 2

mesoderm /'miːzəʊdɜːm/ the 3rd layer of cells in an embryo* from which muscle, bone, connective tissue, etc. develop 3

mesothelium /ˌmesəʊ'θiːlɪəm/ 3

metabolism /mə'tæbəlɪzəm/ the processes by which the body synthesises complex substances from simple ones, and breaks down complex ones to give energy 7

metronidazole /ˌmetrə'naɪdəzəʊl/ 12

micro- small, minute, undersized

microscope /'maɪkrəskəʊp/ 5

mid- middle

miliary /'mɪlɪərɪ/ 10

mitochondrion /ˌmaɪtə'kɒndrɪən/ 3

mole /məʊl/ C

molecule /'mɒlɪkjuːl/; **molecular** (adj.) /mə'lekjələ/ B

monocyte /'mɒnəsaɪt/ 1

morphine /'mɔːfiːn/ 11

motile /'məʊtaɪl/ able to move 12

motion /'məʊʃən/ an emptying of the bowels*; the matter emptied 12

mucosa /mjʊ'kəʊzə/ a mucous* membrane 12

mucous /'mjuːkəs/ of or relating to mucus*; secreting mucus* 3

mucus /'mjuːkəs/ the clear sticky fluid secreted by mucous glands 12

multiple fission /ˌmʌltɪpəl 'fɪʃən/ a series of divisions of the nucleus followed by a division of the body into as many parts as there are nuclei 12

muscle /'mʌsəl/; muscular (adj.) ('mʌskjʊləʳ/ 1

myelomatosis /ˌmaɪələʊmə'təʊsɪs/ a malignant* tumour* of plasma* cells 10

nasal /'neɪzəl/ of or from the nose 10

nausea /'nɔːzɪə, 'nɔːʒə/ a feeling of being about to vomit* 8

necrosis /nek'rəʊsɪs/ the pathologic* death of a group of cells within an organ (producing pus*) 12

needle /'niːdəl/ a hollow sharp-pointed instrument for injection* or aspiration* 11

negligible /'neglɪdʒəbəl/ 7

Neisseria meningitidis /naɪˌsiːrɪə ˌmenɪn'dʒɪtɪdɪs/ 1

nephron /'nefrɒn/ A

nervous /'nɜːvəs/ of or related to nerves 3

neuro- relating to nerves or nervous tissue

neutralise /'njuːtrəlaɪz/ to make a solution neither acid nor alkaline 9

neutrophil /'njuːtrəfɪl/ 4

niacin /'naɪəsɪn/ 7

node /nəʊd/ a small rounded organ 10

nose /nəʊz/ 1

notochord /'nəʊtəkɔːd/ a column* of cells in the embryo* from which the vertebral column develops 12

nucleolus /njuː'kliːələs, - klɪ'əʊləs/ pl. -li /-laɪ/

nucleus /'njuːklɪəs/ pl. nuclei /-klɪaɪ/ 3

obese /əʊ'biːs/ overweight, extremely fat 8

obstetrics /əb'stetrɪks/ the branch of medicine concerning care of women during pregnancy* and childbirth 6

obstruction /əb'strʌkʃən/ a blockage in a hollow vessel, tube or duct* 7

oedema /ə'diːmə/ 7

oesophagus /ɪ'sɒfəgəs/ 1

offspring /'ɒfsprɪŋ/ the children or young produced by two parents or adults 6

-oid like, resembling

-ology a field of study

opiate /'əʊpɪeɪt/ any drug prepared from opium (which relieves pain, but has other effects on the brain + CNS) 11

organ /'ɔːgən/ 1

organic /ɔː'gænɪk/ of or related to organs or to organisms* 11

organism /'ɔːgənɪzəm/ a living thing with different parts combined in an individual able to grow and reproduce* 1

orifice /'ɒrɪfɪs/ an opening, an entrance to a cavity or tube 2

origin /'ɒrɪdʒɪn/ the beginning or starting point of something 3

-osis a process (e.g. osmosis*); a state (e.g. spherocytosis*); a diseased condition of (nephrosis); a disease caused by (e.g. tuberculosis*); an increase in (e.g. leucocytosis)

osmosis /ɒz'məʊsɪs/ the passage of selected molecules through a semipermeable membrane from a dilute* solution into a more concentrated* one 7

osmotic pressure /ɒz,mɒtɪk 'preʃə/ the pressure (developed by osmosis*) which pulls a substance from a dilute* solution into a more concentrated* one C

osmolarity /ˌɒzmə'lærɪtɪ/ C

otolaryngology /ˌəʊtəʊˌlærɪn'dʒɒlədʒɪ/ the study of ear, nose and throat 6

oxytocin /ˌɒksɪ'təʊsɪn/ a hormone* produced by the posterior pituitary gland which stimulates lactation* and the contraction of the uterus in childbirth C

paediatrics /ˌpiːdɪ'ætrɪks/ the branch of medicine concerned with the care of children 6

pain /peɪn/ a disturbed* sensation causing suffering or distress 11

palpation /pæl'peɪʃən/ examination by touch for purposes of diagnosis;

palpate (v.) /pæl'peɪt/ 11

pancreas /'pæŋkrɪəs/ 2

papilla /pə'pɪlə/ pl. papillae /-liː/ A

parasite /'pærəsaɪt/ an organism* that lives on or in another organism (the host*) from which it gets its food 6

parietal /pə'raɪətəl/ 2

partial pressure /ˌpɑːʃəl 'preʃəʳ/ the force exerted by one gas in a mixture of gases 7

particle /'pɑːtɪkəl/ a small portion or piece of a substance B

pass /pɑːs/ to excrete* faeces* or urine 10

pathogen /'pæθədʒən/ an organism* capable of causing disease; **pathogenic** (*adj.*) /ˌpæθə'dʒenɪk/ 12

pathology /pə'θɒlədʒɪ/ the study of the causes, processes and effects of disease; laboratory findings of disease; **pathologic** (*adj.*) /ˌpæθə'lɒdʒɪk/ 6

patient /'peɪʃənt/ a person who is ill and is under medical treatment* 10

pelvis /'pelvɪs/ a basin-shaped cavity (e.g. renal pelvis) 3; the ilium 2

penetrate /'penɪtreɪt/ to enter through the surface of an organ or the wall of a cavity 6

-penia a deficiency of

peptide /'peptaɪd/ a compound of two or more amino acids 9

perforate /'pɜːfəreɪt/ to make a hole in a hollow organ or through the wall of a cavity 12

peri- about, around, near

periosteum /ˌperɪ'ɒstɪəm/ 3

peripheral /pe'rɪfərəl/ 2

peritoneum /ˌperɪtə'niːəm/ the membrane lining the abdominal cavity and surrounding the abdominal organs 3

permeable /'pɜːmɪəbəl/ 1

pethidine /'peθɪdiːn/ 11

pH /ˌpiː'eɪtʃ/ 9

phagocytic /ˌfægəʊ'sɪtɪk/ 1

phalanx /'fælæŋks/ 2

pharmacology /ˌfɑːmə'kɒlədʒɪ/ the study of drugs and their actions 6

pharynx /'færɪŋks/ 3

phrenic /'frenɪk/ 2

physiology /ˌfɪzɪ'ɒlədʒɪ/ the study of the functions of living organisms* and their parts 6

pituitary pɪ'tjuːɪtərɪ/ an endocrine* gland attached to the bottom of the brain 9

-plasm- part of the substance of a cell

plasma /'plæzmə/ 5

Plasmodium falciparum /plæz'məʊdɪəm ˌfælkɪ'pɑːrəm/; **P. vivax** /-'viːvæks/ 6

platelet /'pleɪtlət/ smallest of the solid particles* in the blood; (thrombocyte) B

pleura /'plʊərə/ *pl.* **-rae** /-riː/ the serous membrane lining the thoracic cavity and surrounding the lungs 3

pneumococcus /ˌnjuːmə'kɒkəs/ 1

pneumonia /njuː'məʊnɪə/ inflammation*

of the (alveoli* of the) lungs from infection* 10

-pnoea respiration, respiratory condition

poison /'pɔɪzɛn/ a substance which, even in small quantities, destroys life or seriously disturbs function 7

pole /pəʊl/ one or other of the two ends of a body A

poly- complex; various; excessive

polycythaemia /ˌpɒlɪsaɪ'θiːmɪə/ 7

polymorphonuclear /ˌpɒlɪmɔː'fəʊ'njuːklɪə/ having a nucleus which consists of a number of lobes* attached to each other 1

pore /pɔːr/ a very small opening (on a surface) B

posterior /pɒ'stɪərɪər/ 2

postural drainage /ˌpɒstʃərəl 'dreɪnɪdʒ/ the removal of pus* from the lungs, etc. by use of gravity and the position of the body (to drain a specific area) 11

potential /pə'tenʃəl/ possible, able to be or become 2

pregnant /'pregnənt/ with child, having a child in the uterus; **pregnancy** (*n.*) /'pregnənsɪ/ 7

produce /prə'djuːs/; **production** (*n.*) /prə'dʌkʃən/ 5

prognosis /prɒg'nəʊsɪs/ 10

protein /'prəʊtiːn/ 3

proximal /'prɒksɪməl/ 2

puncture /'pʌŋktʃər/ to make a hole with a pointed instrument 11

purified /'pjʊərɪfaɪd/ freed from foreign matter; made pure 11

pus /pʌs/ a viscous, yellow-green fluid produced by necrosis* (resulting from infection*) 12

pylorus /paɪ'lɔːrəs/ 2

pyramid /'pɪrəmɪd/ 1

pyrexia /paɪ'reksɪə/ fever* 10

pyruvate /paɪ'ruːveɪt/ a salt or ester of pyruvic acid 7

radiography /ˌreɪdɪ'ɒgrəfɪ/ making X-ray photographs of the body 12

radiology /ˌreɪdɪ'ɒlədʒɪ/ the study of radioactive substances, X-rays, etc. and their use in diagnosis* and treatment* 6

radiotherapy /ˌreɪdɪəʊ'θerəpɪ/ the treatment* of disease by radiation 11

reaction /rɪ'ækʃən/ the response to a stimulus* 11

rectum /'rektəm/ 2

relax /rɪ'læks/ to become loose, or less tense 11

renal /'ri:nl/ of the kidney 2

reproduction /ˌri:prə'dʌkʃən/ the process by which an organism* produces more organisms of the same kind; the production of offspring* 12

resistant /rɪ'zɪstənt/ lacking response to a drug, hormone* or treatment* 8

respiration /ˌrespɪ'reɪʃən/ the act of breathing; the physical and chemical processes by which tissues exchange gases; **respiratory** (*adj.*) /rɪ'spɪrətərɪ/ 3

resuscitation /rɪˌsʌsɪ'teɪʃən/ 11

reticulocyte /rə'tɪkjələʊsaɪt/ an immature erythrocyte 5

reticuloendothelial system /rəˌtɪkjələʊˌendə'θi:lɪəl sɪstəm/ all the phagocytic cells of the body (except leucocytes) 5

retina /'retɪnə/ 3

retro- back, behind

rigid /'rɪdʒɪd/; **rigidity** (*n.*) /rɪ'dʒɪdɪtɪ/ 2

ripen /'raɪpən/ to become mature* 5

rod /rɒd/ a thin, straight object 1

rupture /'rʌptʃər/ a forcible breaking or tearing of a part 6

sac /sæk/ a bag-like covering of a natural cavity 3

sacrum /'seɪkrəm/ 2

sagittal /'sædʒɪtəl/ 2

saline /'seɪlaɪn/ (a solution) containing sodium chloride (NaCl) 11

saliva /sə'laɪvə/ the secretions of the salivary glands in the mouth 6

sanatorium /ˌsænə'tɔ:rɪəm/ 10

saturation /ˌsætʃə'reɪʃən/ the dissolving of the maximum possible amount of a substance in a particular solution 7

scalpel /'skælpəl/ 5

Schistosoma haematobium /ˌʃɪstəʊ'səʊmə hi:mə'təʊbɪəm/; **S. japonicum** /-dʒæ'pɒnɪkəm/; **S. mansoni** /-mæn'səʊnaɪ/ 6

schistosomiasis /ˌʃɪstəʊsəʊ'maɪəsɪs/ 6

sclera /'sklɪ:rə/ 3

-scopy visual or other inspection or examination

secrete /sɪ'kri:t/ to produce (by separation from the blood) and release a substance (usually from a gland) 5

sedative /'sedətɪv/ any drug that has a quietening effect on the central nervous system 11

sedimentation /ˌsedɪmən'teɪʃən/ the process by which materials settle to the bottom of a liquid 10

segmentation /ˌsegmən'teɪʃən/ the process of cell division; **segment** (*v.*) /seg'ment/ 6 ·

semi- half

sensitivity /ˌsensɪ'tɪvətɪ/ the degree of change or responsiveness with respect to drugs or other factors 11

serous /'sɪərəs/ 3

serum /'sɪərəm/ the fluid remaining when cells and platelets* are removed from blood 7

shiver /'ʃɪvər/ the shaking of the body to produce heat 6

sieve /sɪv/ B

sigmoid /'sɪgmɔɪd/ 1

sinus /'saɪnəs/ a narrow cavity occurring naturally in the body (e.g. in a bone) or resulting from disease 10

sinusoid /'saɪnəsɔɪd/ like a sinus* 5

site /saɪt/ the place at which something occurs, or the space it occupies B

sore /sɔ:r/ painful, tender 10

species /'spi:ʃi:z/ a specific group of similar individuals 1

spherocytosis /ˌsferəʊsaɪ'təʊsɪs/ the presence in the blood of large numbers of spherical erythrocytes 5

sphincter /'sfɪŋktə/ a muscle surrounding and closing an orifice* 2

sphygmomanometer /ˌsfɪgmɒmə'nɒmətər/ 5

spinal cord /ˌspaɪnl 'kɔ:d/ 3

spiral /'spaɪərəl/ 1

spirillum /spaɪ'rɪləm/ 1

Spirillum volutans /-vɒ'lu:tænz/ 1

spirochaete /'spaɪrəʊki:t/ 1

Spirochaeta stenostrepta /ˌspaɪrəʊ'ki:tə ˌstenəʊ'streptə/ 1

splanchnic /'splæŋknɪk/ relating to, or supplying, the viscera* C

spleen /spli:n/; **splenic** (*adj.*) /'splenɪk/ 2

sputum /'spju:təm/ mucus*, often with pus*, from the air passages 11

squamous /'skweɪməs/ thin and flat 3

sternum /'stɜ:nəm/ 2

stethoscope /'steθəskəʊp/ 5

stimulate /'stɪmjʊleɪt/ to increase the normal activity of an organ or organism* 5

stomach /'stʌmək/ 1

stool /stu:l/ the material excreted from the bowels* 12

stratified /'strætɪfaɪd/ arranged in layers or strata 3

sub- under, beneath, below, less than

sulphonylureas /ˌsʌlfəʊˌnaɪljəˈrɪəz/ 8
sulphuric acid /səlˌfjʊərɪk ˈæsɪd/ 9
superficial /ˌsuːpəˈfɪʃəl/ 2
superior /suːˈpɪərɪəʳ/ 2
suppress /səˈpres/ to hold back; to prevent from functioning 11
supra- upon, above, beyond, exceeding
surgery /ˈsɜːdʒərɪ/ the (study of the) treatment* of injuries* and diseases by operation i.e. doing something to the body with the hands or an instrument 6
sweating /ˈswetɪŋ/ the excretion of a clear fluid onto the surface of the skin 7
symptom /ˈsɪmptəm/ any change in the body or its functions (observed by the patient) which indicates disease* 6
syndrome /ˈsɪndrəʊm/ a group of symptoms* and signs which characterise* a particular disease 8
synthesis (n.) /ˈsɪnθəsɪs/; synthesise (v.) /ˈsɪnθəsaɪz/ 5
syringe /səˈrɪndʒ/ 5
systolic /sɪsˈtɒlɪk/ relating to the contraction* phase of the cardiac cycle 4
taper /ˈteɪpəʳ/ to become smaller towards one end 1
tear /teəʳ/ damage* caused by pulling apart 11
technique /tekˈniːk/ 11
tender /ˈtendəʳ/ painful to the touch or on palpation*; tenderness (n.) /ˈtendənəs/ 11
tension /ˈtenʃən/ (of a gas) the partial pressure* of one gas in a mixture of gases; the state of being stretched 7
testis /ˈtestɪs/ one of the two male reproductive* glands 10
tetany /ˈtetənɪ/ a condition involving sudden involuntary contractions* of muscles 7
therapy /ˈθerəpɪ/ the treatment* of disease* or patients* 11
thiamin(e) /ˈθaɪəmɪn, iːn/ vitamin B₁ 7
thigh /θaɪ/ 2
thirst /ˈθɜːst/ the feeling of a need to drink water; thirsty (adj.) /ˈθɜːstɪ/
thorax /ˈθɔːræks/; thoracic (adj.) /θɔːˈræsɪk/ 2
thrive /θraɪv/ to grow well 12
throat /θrəʊt/ the pharynx 10
thymus /ˈθaɪməs/ 2
thyroid /ˈθaɪrɔɪd/ 2
thyroxine /θaɪˈrɒksɪn-iːn/ 9

tocopherol /tɒˈkɒfərɒl/ vitamin E 7
tolbutamide /tɒlˈbjuːtəmaɪd/ 8
tone /təʊn/ the normal state of tension* of muscles or other parts 11
tonsil /ˈtɒnsəl/ a mass of lymphoid tissue on either side of the back of the mouth 10
toxin /ˈtɒksɪn/ poison*: toxic (adj.) 7
trace /treɪs/ a very small quantity of 7
trachea /trəˈkɪə/ 2
translucent /trænzˈluːsənt/ allowing some light to pass through 12
transverse /trænzˈvɜːs/ 2
treatment /ˈtriːtmənt/ the actions taken to heal* or manage a disease* or patient* 8
triangle /ˈtraɪæŋɡəl/; triangular (adj.) /traɪˈæŋɡjələʳ/ 1
trophozoite /ˌtrɒfəʊˈzəʊaɪt, trəʊ-/ 12
tube /tjuːb/; tubular (adj.) /ˈtjuːbjələʳ/ 1
tubercle /ˈtjuːbəkl/ a small granular* tumour* 10
tuberculin /tjuːˈbɜːkjəlɪn/ a protein derived* from tubercle bacilli 11
tuberculosis /tjuːˌbɜːkjəˈləʊsɪs/ 10
tumour /ˈtjuːməʳ/ any abnormal mass resulting from excessive multiplication of cells 11
ulcer /ˈʌlsəʳ/ a hole in an epithelial surface with an area of necrosis* below 12
ulceration /ˌʌlsəˈreɪʃən/ the process of formation of ulcers 12
uni- one
ureter /ˈjuːrɪtə/ 2
urinary /ˈjʊərɪnərɪ/ relating to urine or to the system for excreting urine 3
urine /ˈjʊərɪn/ the fluid excreted by the kidneys 6
vagus /ˈveɪɡəs/ the 10th cranial nerve C
vascular /ˈvæskjələʳ/ consisting of or containing (blood or lymph) vessels 2
vegetative /ˈvedʒɪtətɪv/ relating to growth and nutrition (feeding) 12
vena cava /ˌviːnə ˈkɑːvə, -keɪvə/ pl. venae cavae /ˌviːniː ˈkeɪviː/ 2
ventilation /ˌventɪˈleɪʃən/ the act or process of supplying fresh air to the lungs or body 8
ventral /ˈventrəl/ 2
vertebra /ˈvɜːtɪbrə/ pl. vertebrae /-iː/ 2
viable /ˈvaɪəbəl/ living; capable of living 12
viscera (pl.) /ˈvɪsərə/ the organs within the 4 main cavities, especially the abdomen; visceral (adj.) 2

126

vital /'vaɪtl/ relating to life 5

vitreous /'vɪtrɪəs/ 3

vomiting /'vɒmɪtɪŋ/ the forcible ejection of the contents of the stomach through the mouth 8

waist /weɪst/ the part of the abdomen between the hips and the ribs 9

wasting /'weɪstɪŋ/ becoming thin; loss of body tissue 8

wound /wuːnd/ a disturbance* or loss of tissue resulting from surgery* or injury* 7

xerophthalmia /ˌzɪərɒfˈθælmɪə/ 7

zygote /'zaɪgəʊt/ 6

Bibliography

AITKEN, J. T., CAUSEY, G., JOSEPH, J., YOUNG, J. Z. *A Manual of Human Anatomy, Vol. 1, Thorax, Abdomen and Pelvis*. Churchill Livingstone, 3rd edn, 1976.

BELL, G. H. et al. *BDS: Textbook of Physiology & Biochemistry*. Churchill Livingstone, 9th edn, 1976.

GREEN, J. H. *An Introduction to Human Physiology*. Oxford Medical Publications, 4th S.I. edn, 1976.

GREEN, J. H. *Basic Clinical Physiology*. Oxford Medical Publication, 2nd edn, 1973.

GREISHEIMER, E. M., WIEDEMANN, M. P. *Pathologic Physiology*. J. P. Lippincott Co., 9th edn, 1972.

HODGKIN, K. *Towards Earlier Diagnosis*. Churchill Livingstone, 3rd edn, 1973.

LUMLEY, J. S. P. et al. *Essential Anatomy*. Churchill Livingstone, 2nd edn, 1975.

MACLEOD, J. (Ed.). *Davidson's Principles and Practice of Medicine*. Churchill Livingstone, 12th edn, 1977.

MACLEOD, J., FRENCH, E. B., MUNRO, J. F. *Introduction to Clinical Examination*. Churchill Livingstone, 1974.

MANSON BAHR, P. E. C. *Tropical Diseases*. Baillière Tindall, 1972.

SODEMAN, W. A., SODEMAN, W. A. *Pathologic Physiology*. W. B. Saunders Co., 5th edn, 1974.

WARWICK, R., WILLIAMS, P. L. (Eds.). *Gray's Anatomy*. Churchill Livingstone, 35th edn, 1973.

WATERHOUSE, J. A. H. *Cancer Handbook of Epidemiology and Prognosis*. Churchill Livingstone, 1974.

WILLIAMS, P. L., WENDELL-SMITH, G. P. *Basic Human Embryology*. Pitman Medical, 1974.

WINGATE, P. *The Penguin Medical Encyclopedia*. Penguin, 1974.

WINTROBE et al (Eds). *Harrison's Principles of Internal Medicine*. Vols. 1 & 2, McGraw Hill, 7th edn, 1974.